Chocolate
Busters

Also by Jason Vale:

The Juice Master's Ultimate Fast Food
Turbo-charge Your Life in 14 Days
Freedom from the Diet Trap: Slim for Life
7lbs in 7 Days: The Juice Master Diet
Juice Master: Keeping it Simple
5lbs in 5 Days: The Juice Detox Diet
The Funky Fresh Juice Book

Chocolate Busters

THE EASY WAY TO KICK IT!

THE JUICE MASTER
JASON VALE
★★★★★

Thorsons

HarperThorsons
An imprint of HarperCollins*Publishers*
1 London Bridge Street
London SE1 9GF

www.harpercollins.co.uk

First published in 2004
This edition 2008

3 5 7 9 10 8 6 4 2

A catalogue record for this book is
available from the British Library

ISBN 978-0-00-716400-4

Printed and bound in Great Britain by
Clays Ltd, St. Ives plc

MIX
Paper from
responsible sources
FSC
www.fsc.org FSC C007454

Contents

I would like to thank all the people who made this book possible. This includes the publisher, editor, proofreader, my dear friends and close family. All of your support has been fully appreciated and I never take any of you for granted. You have all helped to make a difference to the world of all those who read this book and I thank you all.

1

The Truth, The Whole Nut Truth And Nothing But The Truth!

Ahhh, chocolate. Just the word is enough to make the average person melt faster than the cocoa butter itself, which explains why just the thought of giving it up is usually enough to fill the average chocolate lover with a slight degree of apprehension, and for others, out and out panic! However, it doesn't matter how much of the dark stuff you eat, how often you eat it or whether you believe life just wouldn't be worth living without it; the beautiful truth is anyone can find it easy to kick chocolate – even you!

All that's needed for this minor miracle to manifest itself is an *extremely* open mind, the promise that you will read some of this book *every day*, to keep the momentum going, a willingness to follow my guidelines at the end – oh, and plenty of chocolate! Yep, contradiction in terms though it is, please 'feel free' to continue to eat as much chocolate as your little heart desires until you finish the book (and, no, that doesn't mean taking 20 years to finish the book!). If you do that, if you are willing to really open your mind and put your beloved chocolate on the rack, then your break to freedom from one of the most heavily advertised *junkie foods* in the world is as good as guaranteed.

A WOLF IN CHOCOLATE CLOTHING

The truth is, once we have slowly stripped away the many different layers from this cunning chocolate wolf and unwrapped the cold hard truth lurking beneath the glamorous advertising, product placements and seductive glossy packaging – you will never be able to see chocolate in the same light again. Let me make myself clear here: I don't mean you will go off it slightly and cut down a little, no, no, no – I mean once you are able to see this hyped up, sugar-infested drug food for what it really is and not as you've been conditioned to see it, settling down to a bar of the stuff will be about as appealing as plucking your nasal hairs with a fish fork.

For the first time ever the whole business of chocolate is going to get the licking it deserves and by the time you finish this book, unlike with a 'no-chocolate diet' or going on the 'chocolate wagon', you will not only be *happy* not to eat it (a miracle in itself), but also, when you see other people consuming the stuff, far from envying them (or wanting to hurt them severely!) you will actually feel sorry for them.

However, for this seemingly impossible feat to happen, your current perception of this emotionally driven 'food' needs to take a *massive* shift. Fortunately, this will be a piece of cake (not chocolate obviously!). All we need to do is see through the years of brainwashing we've all been subjected to, explode the myths, shatter the illusions, and discover the *correct* knowledge and *unique way of thinking* that will make the whole process of kicking the choccie habit as easy as organic pie!

KNOWLEDGE IS POWER – BUT ONLY OF THE RIGHT KIND!

Now in case you're a 'virgin' to my world of thinking and have yet to indulge in my first book *Freedom from the Diet Trap: Slim for*

Life, I need you to know from the start exactly where I'm coming from. I'm not into doom and gloom, I don't do willpower, I speak plain English and I tell it like it is. Let me be clear, I'm not here to win any literary awards, by golly gosh no, I'm simply here to shake the chocolate world and provide you with the correct knowledge which will enable you to be free to have a *non*-chocolate break if you so choose! And when I say, 'correct knowledge' I don't mean the usual nonsense you get from what I describe as the 'State the Bleeding Obvious Brigade'. You know, the amazing, mind-blowing and life-changing info they come out with, like:

'Chocolate is full of sugar, it's fattening and it's bad for you – if you stopped eating it, you would feel better.'

Not being funny, but 'cover me in cocoa and lick me all over – you don't say!' Or, my favourite expression at times like this, 'No shit, Sherlock!' Please name me one chocolate eater, one 'chocoholic', nay, one living breathing person on this planet who doesn't know that mass-market junkie chocolate is full of sugar and fattening and I'll eat my creme egg. I think it's safe to say that, in terms of stripping this chocolate wolf and helping you to free yourself, members of the 'State the Bleeding Obvious Brigade' banging on about how bad chocolate is for you – or you saying it to yourself – are about as effective as a state-of-the-art cooker at a raw food convention! In reality this kind of approach often has the opposite effect. One of the times people reach for things like chocolate is when they're feeling down, so if someone tells you how ill or fat you can get (or are) because of chocolate, that can make you feel even worse, so what do you do? You say, 'Sod it' and eat more CHOCOLATE!

THERE'S A WAFER THIN LINE BETWEEN LOVE AND HATE

Everyone and their mother knows that mass-market commercial chocolate is bad for you, you don't have to be Inspector Morse to work it out, do you? The problem is, although everyone knows that chocolate is bad and fattening, they also strongly believe it's blooming lovely and has the amazing power to lift our emotions. So what we are dealing with here is what amounts to the ultimate love/hate relationship; the David and Goliath of mental battles. This is why at this stage you will not be entirely sure whether or not you do want to stop eating chocolate altogether. In all probability, you picked up this book to find a way to cut down a little, go on the chocolate wagon for a while – but kick it altogether, like forever? You've got to be off your rocker! This is also why I realize at this stage I'm half your friend and half your enemy:

'Hooray this guy's going to help me kick chocolate!'
'Damn this guy's going to take away my chocolate …
forever – NO WAY!'

It is also why many people who bought the infamous Atkins Diet book only read a small section of it before discarding it to gather dust on the shelf. They were fine up until he pointed out that chocolate was a dreaded carbohydrate and therefore a no-go area. No white bread is fair enough but no chocolate – BOG OFF, ATKINS! Of the millions of Atkins books sold it is estimated that only about 5% of people actually read the whole book and only a small percentage followed it for longer than a week (Jennifer Aniston being one – and don't we know about it!). This is why if you really want to bust your chocolate love/hate affair, it is essential that you do something that most people who buy books of this nature fail to do – read the whole of the book. Every word has been written for a reason and the book is designed, unlike 'pointing out the obvious' methods, to remove this love/hate chocolate tug-of-war by gradually stripping the chocolate industry bare to reveal the truth. Once you see the truth you will find it very hard, if not impossible, to have any desire for chocolate again.

You will notice that in order to achieve this I will be playing the chocolate industry at their own game by repeating certain points over and over again to make certain they stick in your conscious and sub-conscious mind. So if when you're reading this you come across a similar point or you think 'He's said that already', I know – it's on purpose! Repetition is the key to their advertising and emotional hooking success and it is also key to unhooking the emotional attachment to chocolate. It's about time someone used this same approach of repetition to burst the chocolate bubble. Until the chocolate bubble is burst, you've got more chance of finding true freedom from chocolate as you have making a cup of hot cocoa using a chocolate kettle!

The fact that you are reading this book tells me you probably already know this and are fully aware that willpower alone isn't going to cut the cocoa, and lectures on the evils of chocolate are about as helpful as devices such as chocolate patches. (Yes, you haven't misread, there really are chocolate patches, just like nicotine patches, and I'll be covering these beauties in depth later!) The idea behind the willpower method is to give yourself a good talking to about chocolate; make a mental list of all the reasons why you shouldn't have to eat it, then take a deep breath and hang on in there until the craving goes away. There is one slight flaw with this approach:

THE CRAVING GETS WORSE!

And this is why the last thing you need is a lecture on the evils of why you *shouldn't* eat commercially made chocolate. YOU KNOW THAT! What you need is a full understanding of why you *do* eat it.

You need a simple, yet highly effective approach which will not just allow you to see this stuff in its true light; you also need a unique way of thinking that will allow you to Kick The Chocolate … *and be happy about it.* After all, anyone can stop eating chocolate and be miserable about it – I pulled that off on many occasions and I'm sure you've been pretty good at this yourself in the past; all you need is willpower, determination, positive thinking – oh, and being blooming ratty and miserable to boot!

TAKE FLYTE

Let me give you a quick but simple analogy to explain why so many people struggle using this approach. Imagine a house fly trying to get out of a room through a *closed* window. What chance does it have? Ummm, not a jot. But what if the fly had just returned from a positive thinking fly seminar, would it have a better chance then? Of course not! Physics will tell you that no matter how positive, determined or strong-willed the fly is, it will *never* break the glass. Equally, I will tell you and your past experiences should tell you also, positive thinking, determination and a strong will is *not* enough to kick the chocolate – *and be happy about it!* It is, however, always enough to kick the chocolate – *temporarily* – and be blooming miserable about it!

What you need is *not* a pocket full of willpower, a dose of positive thinking or a lecture; all you need is a mind open enough to help remove the many, many layers of conditioning relating to what can only be described as the king of drug foods.

So, without further ado, let us begin our journey into the world of chocolate by stripping off the first layer. I have called chocolate the king of all drug foods, but king wasn't the title it was first given, in fact the title 'king' would almost be an insult. The truth is that from the dawn of time and even today in many societies, chocolate is still widely regarded as …

2

The Food Of The G.O.D.S.

GLOBAL ORGANIZATION OF DRUG-FOOD SUPPLIERS (G.O.D.S.)

Michael Jacobson was the first person to coin the phrase 'junk food' back in 1972. It rocked the 'sweet' world and, just like the tobacco industry, the chocolate industry hit back with claim after claim of why its product wasn't 'junk', but indeed one of the best food sources on the planet (a point I will shatter in depth later). Well, I will agree with them in one respect, commercially made chocolate isn't junk food at all – no, it's 'DRUG FOOD!' If you think the term 'junk food' played havoc with the industry back in 1972, with sweet sales dropping a massive 25%, just imagine what my term of 'Drug Food' will do.

Let's face facts, chocolate is a massive global business and there is just no way the chocolate industry will let this lie. Please don't be surprised if you start to see scientific paper after scientific paper being produced 'proving' why their product is not addictive (in exactly the same way that tobacco companies did for years). After all, they have a lot which needs protecting. In the United Kingdom alone we spend a whopping £4 billion a year on chocolate. That's £65 for every man, woman and child, or to put it another way, 312 oz a year or, to really bring it home, over 22 lb of chocolate per head per year! Now bear in mind this is the 'average'. Many people are consuming far more than this and the figure doesn't include what we buy from duty-free airports and when we are away abroad. An article in the *Daily Mail* a few years ago ran the headline:

'WHY I MUST EAT 200 CHOCOLATE BARS A WEEK'

They were referring to Maureen Young, a self-confessed 'chocoholic' who ate 200 chocolate bars every week for six years. If my calculations are correct that is a cost of *over* £20,000 in just six years! And that's just one person. Maureen, although clearly more 'addicted' than most, isn't the only one bringing in massive revenue for the chocolate industry. Even the average chocolate addict will get through a whopping £15,000 on chocolate in their lifetime. That figure shouldn't really come as any surprise since in Britain at Easter alone we will get through 100 million eggs; that's nearly two chocolate eggs for every person in Britain – 'Jesus!' (well, quite). But, as you may have guessed, we don't lead the world in chocolate consumption, that title is held by the Swiss, who manage just under 28 lbs a year! The US aren't to be left out either – they spend a staggering $14 billion a year on the dark stuff. M&Ms now rank as the world's most popular confection bringing in an amazing $2 billion a year. Let me emphasize that in case you just skipped over it, that is:

TWO BILLION DOLLARS EVERY YEAR JUST ON M&Ms!

M&Ms, although first made in 1940, were virtually unknown in Britain until a few years ago. When we wanted some round brightly-coloured sweets with chocolate centres it appeared that only 'Smarties had the answer' – which is quite funny as Smarties were first produced in 1937, three years before the now mighty

M&Ms. M&Ms are owned by one of the biggest drug-food giants in the world – Mars Inc – a true superpower in the world of chocolate.

Mars Inc is a company that produces enough Fun Size Milky Way every year literally to reach the Milky Way. In fact, the huge amount of those little, sorry, I mean 'fun-size' choc bars, made every year are enough to circle the globe – TWICE! In the UK we buy 17 million Bounty Bars annually, once again a bestselling confectionery made by – yep, you guessed it – Mars Inc. It is no wonder then that the Mars Inc company are the largest sweet manufacturer in the world. What may come as a surprise though is that Mars, in financial terms, are now bigger than McDonald's with an unbelievable $20 billion a year in sales from various interests.

Chocolate, like most products these days, has big guns globalizing the industry. In 1945 there were roughly 6,000 firms producing the stuff. It is estimated that by 2010 that the number will be as low as 150 worldwide. Mars Inc, in my opinion, are the McDonald's and Marlboro of the chocolate world. And just like the fast-food and nicotine trades, the chocolate industry also has its Burger King, Silk Cut, Wendy's, Benson and Hedges, and Wimpy in the forms of Cadbury, Nestlé, Rowntree, Green & Blacks, Lindt, Thorntons and, in the US, Hershey. In fact, in the US if you mentioned Cadbury they would wonder which planet you're from, but say, Hershey and they immediately know what you mean. That's because in the US Hershey are a very big player in the chocolate world – it even boasts its own town! The battle between Mars and Hershey has been going on for years and it echoes that of Pepsi and Coca-Cola, each company battling for number-one spot. At last count, Hershey was winning the US battle, but, by the time you read this, in the cut-throat, back-stabbing, idea-pinching world of chocolate, that could have easily changed. However, whatever the chocolate company, just like their nicotine, caffeine and fast-food cousins, each, on a financial front, are doing just fine and dandy thank you very much. And this is why chocolate is now one of the most traded commodities in the world, and to the villagers on small farms in places such as West Africa, and on plantations owned by wealthy land barons in other parts of the world, cocoa is as important to the economies of these countries as oil is to the Middle East.

Cadbury, Britain's leader in the land of the chocolate, aren't too far behind. Despite their 'local brand' impression – Cadbury are a major global player. Two billion bars of Cadbury's chocolate are bought every year. If just the creme eggs it produces each year were stacked on top of each other they would be 900 times higher than Mount Everest, and if the Crunchies eaten in the same length of time were lined up they would stretch from Birmingham to Bangkok. On top of that, just like Hershey in the States, Cadbury even has its own town – Bournville, or as they like to describe it, Cadbury World.

Chocolate has also been written about in some of the most famous children's stories ever told, from *Charlie and the Chocolate Factory* to the modern-day phenomenon which is Harry Potter. Major blockbuster films have not just featured it but have even been based on and named after it – *Chocolat* being the obvious example. There are few items in the world that do not have a chocolate version of them somewhere. You can get chocolate televisions, chocolate typewriters, chocolate hats, chocolate houses, chocolate cigarettes, chocolate body paint, chocolate love toys (I didn't say all chocolate was bad!) and there is even a place that will make an exact replica of your good self carved entirely from chocolate!

It has been linked to every emotion we possess and the Global Organization of Drug-food Suppliers (GODS) have managed, through clever advertising, to make us believe it can *genuinely* help our moods, act as a catalyst to the land of the bliss and, more recently, that it is actually good for us (this point will be covered in depth a little later). They have also managed to make it perfectly normal to start children on this stuff from an extremely early age. In fact, they have so brainwashed and conditioned us that if we *don't* give children chocolate, especially if they have been 'good', we are the ones who are seen as the bad guys!

So how have we reached the stage where so many people believe that life wouldn't be the same without a mass of drug-like substances entering their bloodstream on a regular basis? Why do we automatically think of chocolate when Valentine's Day comes around, or Mother's Day, or Christmas Day, or Easter Day, or a birthday – or, let's face it, any day? Why do we continue to eat this stuff even though we nearly always feel sick and 'Oh, I wish I hadn't done that' afterwards? Why is it so strongly linked to love, comfort, joy and, of course, PMS? Why does it seem to take such an emotional hold unlike any other 'food' on the planet?

THE ANSWER COULD LIE IN A BROWNIE

A Derren Brownie to be precise (well, Derren Brown actually). Anyway, I don't know if you've seen this guy, but he is known as a 'mind control expert' and he is exceptionally brilliant at what he does. I watched a programme of his once where he took two advertising 'geniuses', people who prided themselves on being the best in the business; able to come up with *unique* ideas super-fast. Derren Brown arranged transport for these men to meet him in a hotel room. Once there he unveiled a large stuffed bear as their brief. Yes, they had to do an advertising campaign for a taxidermist and they had just half an hour to come up with it. Derren Brown placed a stuffed cat on top of a sealed envelope. He told them under no circumstances were they to touch the envelope. When he returned half an hour later the two quick-thinking advertising gurus had indeed managed to come up with a catchy advertisement. Now please bear in mind they had a blank page and could have put just about anything. As you may have guessed, when Derren asked them to open the envelope he had predicted the exact logo and, as near as damn it, advertising slogan as the two guys. At first they tried to dismiss it (I think their pride was a tad hurt) but in the end they had no explanation as to how on earth he could have predicted their choice of thoughts.

IT'S WHAT YOU'RE NOT CONSCIOUS OF THAT GRABS YOU

The reason why he was able to predict their thoughts was simply because he had already placed them there. What I'm saying is that the advertisement and slogan were never their idea at all – it had been cleverly planted in their subconscious mind on the cab journey over. How? Quite simply by placing both the ad and slogan many times at several stages along the route. For example, at one point the taxi stopped at a crossing and about 20 people, each with t-shirts printed both back and front with the ad and slogan, crossed the road. The ad and slogan were shown many times in this manner throughout their short journey. Derren even arranged that as they entered the hotel, a man holding a newspaper would be leaving. And what was the headline on the paper? Yep – the ad and slogan. So what the hell has that got to do with chocolate? Well, bucket loads actually.

IN THE HANDS OF THE GODS

Up till now, your buying and consumption of chocolate literally has been in the hands of the GODS. They are the 'mind controllers' of the chocolate world and it's their job to make sure that you continue to buy, buy, buy. Like our two advertising people, what you believe to be *your* idea – to buy chocolate in this case – is often anything but. The hard reality is the GODS have been planting images and catchy slogans throughout your journey through life with the sole purpose of getting you conditioned to buy the stuff – most of the time without even knowing what made you do it. This is why **a massive 90% of all chocolate sales are what is known as 'point-of-sale' or 'impulse' buys**. Yes, surprising as it may sound, according to the chocolate companies themselves only 10% of chocolate sales are actually pre-planned (ie, gifts for Mother's Day, saying, 'I love you' and so on); the rest are made on 'the spur of the moment' – or are they?

The 90% of sales apparently made on impulse are at times such as when you are standing in a queue at a supermarket and just happen to see a glossy packet containing chocolate; or when you are waiting for a train and you hear the cry of glass-imprisoned chocolate bars screaming at you to set them free; or when you stop for petrol and grab a bar when paying – you know that sort of thing. However, the cocoa seeds of purchase must have already been sown some time *prior* to the moment of buying. Think about it, would a non-smoker ever buy cigarettes 'on the spur of the moment'? Would they ever ask for some simply because they happen to have bought some petrol? Would they hear the loud cries from nicotine packets as they begged for freedom from their glass prisons on station platforms? No, of course not! If you don't smoke you don't buy them, no matter what impulsive mood you are in; smokers buy cigarettes because they are *already* conditioned to smoke – in exactly the same way that you are *already* mentally and physically conditioned to eat chocolate.

In truth the conditioning has been going on ever since you were old enough to say, 'The Milky Bars Are On Me' and has been going strong throughout your life. Product placement after product placement, billboard after billboard, TV campaign after TV campaign, sponsorship after sponsorship, even government literature cleverly designed to plant the idea that life is just simply more fun with a 'boost' or 'treat' of chocolate and all those who don't indulge are clearly boring no-hope health freaks who are obviously a few cocoa beans short of a full pod!

There is no question that placing chocolate at the checkouts of supermarkets, newsagents and petrol stations plays a massive role in their sales. It is also true that many people wouldn't buy half as much if they didn't have it shoved in their face at every opportunity. However, the point is that you have already been conditioned to eat it for this kind of product placement to have the desired effect. Recently there have been calls for this kind of product placement to be banned, especially where it is aimed at children, but I think there is more chance getting run over by a giant Easter egg than this ever happening.

GREAT CHOCOLATE SMOKES ALIVE

The chocolate companies, just like the nicotine boys and girls, are true masters of the emotional hook, not just on a mental level but also at a physical one. Get the two right and BOOM – you've got one almighty addictive winner, a lifelong customer and, of course, several penthouses in Malibu! In fact, the similarities between the tobacco and chocolate industries are more than a little spooky and go way beyond the striking similarity between the Silk Cut colour and that of Cadbury Dairy Milk (have you noticed that?).

Both cigarettes and chocolate have colourful glossy packets, both have used words like 'satisfying', 'lift' and 'light' in their advertising campaigns, both have role models such as the 'Marlboro Man' and the 'Milky Bar Kid', both have regal or 'out of this world' names, such as 'Royal' and 'Super Kings' in the cigarette world and 'Mars', 'Milky Way' and 'Galaxy' in the chocolate world. In fact, both even have names with Death in the title. There is a brand of cigarettes called 'Death' (how nice) and a (how can you describe it?) big blob of chocolate called 'Death By Chocolate'. Both chocolate and cigarettes have been given to troops in World War II, both have gone to considerable lengths to prove their product is not just safe but has incredible health benefits, and both have one person in common – Philip Morris. Philip Morris not only owns the world's leading cigarette company, Marlboro, but has recently started buying chocolate companies. They even beat the mighty American chocolate company Hershey to acquiring Freia Marabou, a Norwegian chocolate company with a strong presence in Scandinavia. On top of that, they also once owned and, I understand, still have plenty of shares in Kraft Jacobs Suchard: a company which produces Terry's All Gold and perhaps the most instantly recognizable chocolate in the world – Toblerone. Toblerone's slogan was always 'Out On Its Own', but next time you have a triangular-shaped choccie, spare a thought for the extra money you're ploughing into Philip Morris's pocket, helping to make sure that, on a financial front, they are truly 'out on their own'. The coincidences don't stop there either. Even Philip Morris's 'Marlboro Man' was created by Leo Burnett, the same person who came up with the much-loved Uncle Ben character – owned by Master Foods, part of the Mars company.

Such is the power of Philip Morris that they have managed with Toblerone to do what the makers of 'Sunny Delight' did with their product. One minute it wasn't there, the next every shelf was packed with the stuff. Some of the biggest sales for Philip Morris come from duty-free shops in the airports of the world. You can't but fail to notice the large, gold-wrapped, glossy boxes of … chocolate! Yes, haven't you noticed that now Toblerone not only has the same colour wrappings as Benson and Hedges cigarettes, but it has also grown just a bit in size? Have you also noticed the shelf space when these massive bars of Toblerone have been found? Have a look next time you're in a duty free – at first glance you would think there is no other chocolate on the planet except Toblerone. And be aware that getting this kind of shelf space is no easy feat – you need more contacts than Specsavers to pull it off … oh, and flipping great wedges of cash too! This is because of the 90% 'point-of-sale' factor – it's all about being seen.

I always suspected there must be some link between the two ever since I used to buy chocolate cigarettes – when I was just seven years old! If they can make chocolate cigarettes legal for children, I really wouldn't put anything past them. Forrest Mars was even once a travelling salesman … for Camel cigarettes! It was also partly due to cigarettes that the Mars company grew the way it did. According to Forrest Mars, it all started with a simple suggestion to his father Frank, 'Why don't you manufacture something like Camel cigarettes?' And the rest is history.

There is one other similarity between the two which I forgot to mention – both cigarettes and chocolate can be highly addictive. The chocolate companies, however, like their cigarette industry cousins, will naturally deny this until we are blue in the face, but somehow I don't think it's disputable.

WHAT IS ADDICTION ANYWAY?

Put simply, addiction is a mental and/or physical hook, hence the expression 'hooked'. Addiction is an emotion and the emotion is fear. Any substance which creates the fear that life wouldn't be the same without it, that you wouldn't be able to cope with and/or enjoy your life the same way without it, is an addictive drug. So does mass-market chocolate fall into this category? You'd better bet your chocolate bottom it does.

Now clearly addiction has its levels and I realize that not everyone who eats chocolate is like Maureen Young (the woman who used to get through 200 bars of chocolate a week), but the fact that so many people are buying this book because they want to stop eating it is surely proof of its addictive nature. I mean, even if you loved them, you wouldn't need to buy a book entitled The Simple Way to Stop Eating Sardines if you wanted to stop eating sardines, would you? There aren't any 'sardine patches' or organizations such as Sardine-olic Anonymous are there? Yet there are 'chocolate patches', there are people who run their lives with a Chocoholics Anonymous way of thinking, and there are thousands of people spending God knows how much on therapies such as acupuncture and hypnotherapy in an attempt to free themselves of their craving for chocolate. If it were their genuine choice to eat chocolate, then surely they could simply make a genuine choice not to eat it – couldn't they? So is it possible that some Derren Brown-like activities have been at work to make people believe it is their choice when really they have been mentally hooked?

With that in mind, I think the addiction part is pretty clear. Fortunately, 99% of the hook is mental, created by years and years of clever marketing; the actual physical withdrawal (if you can even call it that) you will simply not notice. However, like most addictions, let's not underestimate the power of the emotional hook because it is this which drives the fear.

FALSE EMOTION THAT APPEARS REAL

The fact is the GODS, through clever emotional advertising, emotional conditioning *and* mood-altering chemicals (yes, there is a physical part), have managed to create a powerful and emotionally driven food. As such, people become mentally and physically 'attached' and in many cases getting rid of chocolate proves as difficult as ending a relationship; they literally feel fear at letting go and so are 'hooked'. Luckily, the emotions created by the marketing and the chemicals are all false, they just *appear real.* After all, what on earth can possibly happen to you if you do stop eating chocolate? Your heads are hardly going to explode and you are certainly not going to starve. So any fears you may have about getting rid of chocolate from your life are completely false. That said, when something *appears* real it then *is* real to that person.

The only way to kick the chocolate – *and be happy about it* – is fully to shatter those fears and see this stuff and its pushers for what they really are. With that in mind, let's really start to unwrap the industry by taking a long hard look behind the advertising and conditioning before we unwrap the many layers of the product itself.

One of the most famous lines with the word Mars in the title has got to be that from a very insightful John Gray – *Men are from Mars, Women are from Venus* – but it's still not a patch on the most successful one ever used. I don't think there's a single person, in the UK at least, who doesn't know …

3

A Mars A Day Helps You Work, Rest And Play

One thing is undisputed – advertising works, especially when you are dealing in an addictive substance. And the chocolate big boys and girls spend an absolute fortune making sure their particular message stays in the forefront (and the depths) of our easily manipulated minds. Over and over and over again they beam the same messages into our computer-like brains, making certain that we download the information into our hard drives. Mars alone spends $400 million a year advertising in the US, Cadbury spends a whopping £250 million just in the UK. Each chocolate company does their utmost to make sure we never forget that 'Nothing Satisfies Like A Snickers', that when you have a break you should most certainly 'Have A Kit Kat' or if things get on top of you, you should 'Take It Easy With Cadbury's Caramel'. Each company cleverly links our emotions, sporting abilities and even good health with their product. And each company makes sure that we believe the hype.

MARS SPONSORS MARATHON

Mars paid $2 million for the worldwide rights to the Rolling Stones song 'Satisfaction' to help promote the company's leading product – Snickers. But that is small change compared with the $5 billion they forked out to be the official sponsor of the 1984 Olympics. They also are a major sponsor in the football World Cup and, seemingly, will not miss any opportunity to link their product to something exciting and, ironically, sporty. This point was hammered home to me when I saw a friend of mine running on a treadmill in my local gym dressed as a Mars Bar. It turned out that Mars was sponsoring him to run the London marathon, a point which would have been made a lot funnier if the chocolate bar Marathon wasn't now called Snickers! It took him over five hours to complete the race with buckled knees in what amounted to a Mars boiler suit. He explained how all the way around the streets of London on one of the hottest marathon days in history, he heard rendition after rendition of 'A Mars A Day Helps You Work, Rest And Play' – how's that for illustrating the power of advertising! I think Mars got their money's worth – not only was their big bar in full view of the millions of spectators, but it was also featured on BBC TV, a broadcasting company which prides itself on the fact that they don't advertise! And what sort of pay did he get for nearly knackering his knees for life and giving the GODS massive exposure? Forty-eight Mars Bars! Unlike my friend, Mars are in my opinion just pretending it's all for charity, pretending it's all for the greater good, but in truth it's probably all bullshit. After all, the advertising opportunities at these sort of events must be the primary motivation for sponsoring them anyway. I'm not just picking on Mars here; most of the big chocolate companies are up to this sort of thing, especially the UK's biggest brand of chocolate, Cadbury. In Spring 2003, 'The Nations Favourite' (their words not mine) launched a £9m campaign to persuade children to buy 160m of their chocolate bars in exchange for sports equipment for their schools – yes, SPORTS EQUIPMENT! They called the scheme – 'Cadbury Get Active' and said their initiative would 'help to tackle obesity'. They managed to do this through the Youth Sport Trust and it was endorsed by the Labour minister of sport Richard

Caborn. Imagine if Benson & Hedges decided to encourage children to smoke in return for donating some money towards cancer research; would the health minister allow that as it will 'help a good cause'? Cadbury even managed to get Paula Radcliffe to back the 'Get Active' marketing scheme. Paula is not just an athlete, but a super athlete. At the time of writing this book, she reigns supreme in the long-distance running world, almost breaking a new record every time she sets foot on a track. The link here is clear, eat this stuff and it will help you be a supreme athlete; it will give you energy; it will keep you going; it may even make you a star! Mind you, at least finding out that chocolate companies sponsor sports stars has exposed what Linford Christie might have had in his lunch box – two creme eggs and a king-size Mars bar!

Cadbury not only recruit lean athletic stars to link the image of sport and health with a product full of fat and sugar, but they also sponsor one of the most watched television shows in the UK – Coronation Street. Their aim here is to make sure that the relaxed, end-of-the-day, put-your-feet-up feeling gets associated with their product. Does it work? I should coco! The people who make the decisions to spend millions advertising and sponsoring sports events or TV shows aren't stupid – they more than know what they are doing. They know that if they can link a positive emotion or 'feel good' factor to their product they're onto a winner and, boy oh boy, are they good at it?

'The Sweetest Things On Earth Come From Mars'
                         (US Advertising slogan for Mars in the 1960s)

Every time you see a chocolate ad, hear a slogan, see a piece of chocolate cleverly placed in a film or catch a glimpse of a glossy wrapper out of the corner of your eye when at a theme park such as Disney World, you can be sure that months of planning and board meetings went into making it happen. Advertising and marketing are a science and the not-so-mad professors are paid massive amounts to come up with catchy slogans and think up ingenious ideas that will lure you in and get you emotionally hooked. Bill Suhring, ex-marketing man at Mars and creator of the slogan above, was paid a basic salary of $35,000 a year (back in 1968!) to head marketing at Mars' arch-rivals Hershey. To put this in perspective, even the president of the chocolate giant Hershey didn't make that sort of money back then. Marketing was, and is, taken very seriously and in the cut-throat Willy Wonka world of chocolate, anything goes.

SWEET FA – FALSE ADVERTISING

In the UK there is a body called the 'Advertising Standards Authority' (ASA), made up of individuals whose sole purpose is to make sure that the claims made in advertisements are true, accurate and not misleading in any way. With that in mind, doesn't it make you wonder how slogans such as '… Makes You Work, Rest and Play' or 'Gives You A Boost' pass the strict advertising rules, especially when in a recent advert I wrote for a juice extractor, I wasn't allowed to use the word 'healthy' in it – and that was for fresh fruits and vegetables! Somebody did once take Mars to court over their 'A Mars A Day …' slogan, claiming it was completely false and that no one product can possibly help you work, rest and play. I suppose arguing that work and rest are two complete opposite situations and it would have to be some kind of miracle product to act as a relaxant one minute and a stimulant the next. A good argument I would have thought, but guess who won?

Yep – Mars!

'THINKING ABOUT YOUR CHOCOLATE ... THINKING ABOUT YOUR TASTE'

One of the all-time chocolate mind-manipulation adverts has to be that of the 1988 advertising campaign for Cadbury's Dairy Milk. The advert showed photographs of normal everyday images being transformed into Cadbury's chocolate. The campaign was, according to Cadbury's own literature, '... built on the thought of chocolate becoming a compulsion, which a person cannot get out of their mind ...' They then explain that, 'running through was the haunting slogan ... "Thinking about your chocolate ... thinking about your taste."' As the campaign grew in momentum many different scenarios manifested. One showed a man in his convertible car and, in his mind, the badge on the front turns into Cadbury's chocolate; another featured a photographer with a glamorous model whose shimmering purple gown turns into a bar of chocolate. The idea of the ad was to repeat the message 'Thinking about your chocolate ... thinking about the taste' over and over again, until we actually did. They want you to have a 'compulsion' for their drug food and they want you to 'not get it out of your mind' – it is this which brings in sales. I wouldn't be surprised if at some point someone uses Kylie Minogue's 'Can't Get You Out Of My Head' and attaches it to their product or food. This type of ad not only manipulates the mind, but it also prays on our emotions. In fact, the biggest trick of all in advertising is to find a subtle way to link feel-good emotions to their products, and the chocolate industry really do reign supreme in this field.

TCI FRIDAY

Certain days of the week are synonymous with certain feelings, and none more so than Friday. Ever since we started school, Friday has had a different feeling to any other day – it has what can only be described as 'That Friday Feeling'. It's a feeling that was quickly exploited by the chocolate industry. So now you don't have to thank that fact you've been paid, or that the week is over, or that you can let your hair down that it's Friday – NO, now you can 'Thank Crunchie It's Friday'! Not only have they cleverly managed to link this sugar-infested, sorry, I mean 'Honey-Combed' product with a feeling that's got not a jot to do with Crunchie at all, but they also managed to reinforce the message with the musical lyrics which accompanied the ad. If you can't recall it, allow me:

'I'm so excited, and I just can't hide it, I know, I know, I know, I know, I know that I want you – want you.'

A Derren Brown moment if ever I heard one! And if one Friday afternoon you do find yourself feeling good and just happen to 'spontaneously' reach for a Crunchie – WHAM, they've got you! The minute your brain links *that* feeling with *that* product it will search for it again, perhaps on a cold, bleak, boring Tuesday afternoon, for example.

From the first moment your brain makes a positive connection between chocolate and emotion you're in trouble … and they know it.

This is why Mars has recently gone one better than the Crunchie gang by creating a slogan and a £2 million ad campaign that manages to link the product to just about *any* wonderful and joyous emotion. Yes, gone are the days where 'A Mars A Day Helps You Work, Rest And Play', now we have a product which produces 'Pleasure You Can't Measure'. Yep, somehow this little mind-twister slipped past the people at trading standards. Billboard after billboard depict pictures and captions of moments in our life where the pleasure just cannot be measured. 'Your First Kiss' reads one, 'Weekends' says another. Ad after ad depicting some silly and many wonderful moments that you truly want to recapture, especially when you're lonely or having a bad day. This is why there's hardly a person on the planet who, when they're feeling down says, 'Bugger it, I'm having a grape!', but there are thousands of people who say, 'Sod it, life's too short' and reach for some chocolate. People don't reach for grapes for one reason – the British grape industry hasn't conditioned them to eat grapes as a response to emotion – and, oh yes, grapes aren't full of unnatural drug-like substances!

REAL CHOCOLATE – FALSE FEELINGS

In an advert for Cadbury's Dairy Milk, one of the bestselling chocolate bars in Britain, we see a young boy playing Saturday morning football. The picture shows all the dads cheering on their boys, and one woman, his mother, doing her best to join in. As the game ends we see the boy looking sadly at all the dads. Then his mum hands him some Dairy Milk and as she does so, the caption appears, 'You're a great striker son.' His sad face turns into a loving smile and as he looks up to her the caption reads, 'You're a great Dad, Mum.' The ad then finishes with the slogan, 'Real Chocolate – Real Feelings'. How's that for pulling on your emotional heart strings? How's that for linking massive feelings to their product. How they get away with this blatant hogwash is a mystery to one and all. I suppose the biggest irony of this ad is that the combination of drug-like ingredients which go into making a chocolate bar like this creates *false* chocolate – *false* feelings.

AND ALL BECAUSE THE LADY LOVES ...

Then, of course, you have the ads for chocolate which focus on another couple of our most powerful emotions – love and gratitude, often linking the two beautifully. When it comes to gratitude, Cadbury once again get star billing with their incredibly

successful 'Thank You Very, Very Much' Cadbury's Roses campaign.
When it comes to love, they're all at it, jumping on the back of
history. Back in the days when it was believed chocolate was a
'cure all', drinking chocolate was known as a 'potion of love'. The
Aztecs regarded chocolate as an aphrodisiac and Emperor
Montezuma was said to down a golden goblet full of the rich,
brown liquid each time he entered his harem of 500 beautiful
women. Call me Mr Cynical, but somehow I think his sexual ability
just might have had something to do with 500 naked women in his
room and not so much the drinking chocolate! But despite
chocolate doing absolutely nothing for your sexual prowess and
being gooey, sticky and often sickly, chocolates in general are now
an accepted way of saying, 'I love you.'

Do you remember 'All because the Lady Loves Milk Tray' or 'Do
you love anyone enough to give them your last Rolo?' or how
about, 'See the face you love light up with Terry's All Gold.' Now
call me Mr Party Pooper, but this is hardly a good way to express
your love is it? 'Happy Valentines my sweet, here's something that
will cause you to feel fat and hate yourself' – well, cheers! I wonder
if the advert would have had the same pull if the slogan ran, 'See
the face you love blow up with Terry's All Gold'. Perhaps not!

ONLY THE CRUMBLIEST ...

There is, however, one human drive which is perhaps stronger than
any other – SEX! Whether it's politically correct or not to say so,
the fact remains that sex sells, it always has done and always will.
Now there's a fine line between sex and love, but unlike Milk Tray,
Rolo or Terry's All Gold, Cadbury's Flake cannot fool us into
thinking it's all about love. No, if we put our honest heads on for a
second, Flake equals sex, or DIY sex if we're really getting to the
nitty-gritty. One of the first ever ads to feature Flake ran the
advertising slogan, 'By Yourself? Enjoy Yourself' – and that, was in

the 1950s! Yes, it's all about coming home, running a bath, getting naked and blocking out the stresses of the world by simulating oral sex with a chocolate bar. This isn't my imagination either; it was more than a little deliberate. Thomas Krygier, one of the advertising gurus in charge of the Flake ad campaign, says they deliberately looked for innocent-looking women to front their ads. In his words, 'You wouldn't expect her to give a blow job!' The idea, of course, was to illustrate that even innocent-looking people can be naughty and that chocolate had always been seen as 'naughty but nice'. This idea perhaps reached its climax when the soul singer Joss Stone became the first famous person ever to advertise Flake.

The emotional hook is what they want – what they need – and it is what keeps them turning over billions. In business terms, they want what is known as 'the lifetime value of a customer'. That's why they can spend millions advertising something which costs about 30p. It's the repetition they want and what better way to guarantee that than the emotional hook. This is why pop bands, which already have an emotional hook with their huge child fan base, are paid millions of pounds by companies such as Cadbury. The priceless emotional hook has already been established. What's more, the children also trust the band, so if the pop group eats or drinks it, the children believe it must not only be cool but also good. This is why getting Harry Potter signed up was such an incredible coup for our friends at Mars and Coca-Cola. Harry Potter is a modern-day phenomenon and if they can get Harry to eat a Mars and drink a Coke … that really would be magic!

As I'm sure you're starting to realize, the chocolate industry will use just about any emotion, any situation to give the impression that their particular chocolate will help in some way. They are trying, very successfully, to build a relationship between you and the product. The bond ends up being so great that even a simple name change, let alone giving it up, can cause people to get a little touchy.

'It's a Marathon, for Christ's Sake!'

See what I mean? Uniformed branding is extremely important to the big players in the chocolate world, and it means they can achieve global sponsorship and brand familiarity worldwide. This was the problem Mars had sponsoring in the 1984 Olympics, they quickly realized they didn't have uniformity. It was then they set out to make sure that all chocolate bars in the US would be instantly recognizable across the globe. Hence Marathon becoming Snickers, Treets becoming M&Ms, etc. Once they have uniformity they know their job will be made much, much easier in the future.

The loyalty to brands is so strong that instead of bringing out brand-new chocolate bars, which can involve incredible risk, years from idea to birth, and millions in cash building a new relationship, they simply add different ingredients and produce a different version of an already named brand. This is why we get many different versions of M&Ms and products such as Milky Way Dark and *Snow* Flake.

Generating a following and brand loyalty is something the chocolate industry seemingly will go to any lengths to achieve. Not long after the collapse of the former Soviet Union, Mars used huge amounts of emotional advertising to achieve what the press called 'the Snickerization of Russia'. Months prior to introducing the Russians to their first 'hit' of this legal drug food, they carefully manipulated their minds, not just by erecting massive billboards showing their glossy packaged products, but also dangling the emotional hook by throwing a Christmas party for disadvantaged children – sounds generous, until you understand the motives behind the move. The party included a rock party for 4,000 teens, which attracted large TV coverage. TV coverage in a country with only one or two channels does nothing other than link the Mars brand to 'party mood' and generosity. On top of this they ran an advertising campaign which used the theme:

'All the World Loves M&Ms'

A statement which is untrue, but it was still allowed to be used.
The combination of the advertising and 'generosity' meant that the
Russians had been mentally teased on a massive scale. So much so
that on 4 January 1990, a quarter of a mile of Russians, pockets
stuffed with roubles, police at the ready, queued to get their first
taste of the West. Mars sold more than 20 tons of chocolate in just
two days, and this was with a restriction on how much each person
could buy! In a very short space of time Mars had achieved its
objectives – to create an emotional hook to the brand before
supplying them with the chemical 'hit'.

However, the chocolate advertising boys and girls don't always
get it right when dabbling in politics to help sell their wares. The
not-so-forward-thinking Cadbury marketing people in India
thought they would try to sell more chocolate by playing on the
biggest issue facing the world's largest democracy – Kashmir. This
is an issue which continues to threaten to plunge India and its
neighbour, Pakistan, into nuclear war. Newspaper advertisements
for the Temptations range of chocolate depicted a map of Kashmir
alongside the riddle: 'I'm good. I'm tempting. I'm too good to share.
What am I? Cadbury's Temptations or Kashmir?' As soon as it came
out, as you can well imagine, waste matter hit the fan and the
company were forced to apologize. Mr Vinod Tawde, leader of the
Bharatiya Janata Party said, 'Why use an emotive issue like
Kashmir to promote products?' The answer is very clear – because
it works … usually! They want to stir up emotions – that's the
whole point. They want people to take notice. Unfortunately for
them this one backfired, but they're usually spot on.

ET – EXTRA TURNOVER

Although advertising and sponsorships are clear winners, they pale into complete insignificance when compared to good product placement. If you can get a picture of a Milky Way or Flake in a blockbuster film like James Bond, you've done well, but get Bond to eat it on screen and WHAM – you have a winner! With that in mind, please spare a thought for Mars who turned down Steven Spielberg's offer for M&Ms to be ET's favourite sweet in one of the biggest grossing films of all time. Perhaps they didn't think the film would ever catch the public imagination – dough! Instead, the contract went to Mars' rival, Hershey and their sweet named Reese's Pieces. Although not a chocolate product, there are few who believe Reese's Pieces were not designed to go head to head with Mars' bestselling product, M&Ms – they even look similar. Jack Dowed was Hershey's marketing man at the time and there is just no way that he or anyone at Hershey could have envisaged just what a coup getting the ET gig was. Nothing like that had ever been done before and although the thought seems crazy now, at the time it was a massive $ lm risk. Bear in mind that Dowed made the deal without seeing a script or an image of the alien, and with the knowledge that although Spielberg had been successful with films such as *Duel* and *Jaws*, his previous film *1941* starring John Belushi completely bombed. However, according to Dowed himself it turned out, 'The biggest marketing coup in history.' With such emotional triggers proclaiming that Reese's Pieces were 'ET's favourite sweet' being plastered everywhere, and with cinemas all over the country putting the product in prime buying spots in their display cabinets, sales shot through the roof. Distributors reported as much as a tenfold increase during the 14-day film launch.

THE ULTIMATE CHOCOLATE RAPPER

Mars may have missed out there, but in the late 1990s and early 2000s, they struck lucky as the biggest-selling rap artist of all time adopted the street name of one of their bestselling chocolates – M&Ms. Now, you may think I've made a huge mistake here and that it's not M&M but Eminem. In fact, when this incredible rapper started out his name really was M&M. The cost to Mars for this association – sweet nothing!

IT'S ALL 'OK' IT SEEMS

Because good product placement has the power to reap such incredible financial rewards, it appears the chocolate companies will stop at nothing to get a shot of some celebrity eating their product into a magazine or newspaper. A few years ago *OK* magazine paid Anthea Turner and Grant Bovey an undisclosed six-figure sum for the exclusive wedding picture rights. It is something which Anthea Turner now deeply regrets, and for a very good reason. As part of the 'exclusive' deal, *OK* was to sell-on just *one* photo of the happy day to the UK daily newspapers. Unfortunately for them, the photograph *OK* chose to sell to the newspapers was one of the couple eating a chocolate bar. The magazine thought it was more than OK to have a deal with Cadbury. Their job was to make sure they got a good picture of Anthea and Grant eating one of Cadbury's new chocolate bars named 'Snowflake'. They managed to get their prize picture by persuading Anthea and Grant – at the end of a long day – to pose for one last 'tongue-in-cheek' photo.

Despite what so many people think, the truth is that neither Anthea nor Grant was paid a penny by Cadbury and the deal was all *OK*'s doing. Not only did it ruin what should have been happy memories of a special day, but it also lost Anthea her job as a television presenter after the slagging off she got in the press, thus causing her to fall out of favour with the 'we love Anthea' British public. Never mind, though – *OK* got their picture and Cadbury was laughing all the way to the bank with one of the biggest product placement scoops in recent British history.

KIND 'ER' NO SURPRISE REALLY

I think it's fair to say then that when it comes to marketing, the chocolate big guns will do just about anything to help sell their wares, and in an industry not renowned for its scruples, it's no surprise that their main marketing focus seems to be aimed at those whose brains are most susceptible to the emotional hook – children! Unlike the tobacco companies, who at least had to pretend they weren't targeting kids (although that's hard to believe when you see Joe Camel), the chocolate industry can do it with impunity.

Research carried out by the Foods Standards Agency found a direct link between overweight children and TV advertising. This may be pretty obvious to you and me, especially when you think that food is by far the most commonly advertised product category and given the four 'food' products dominating this advertising are 'soft' drinks, pre-sugared cereals, confectionery snacks (including chocolate) and fast-foods, but the FDA needed a full study to see what was happening. As of October 2003 the top two food products advertised to children were for chocolate, the number one spot being held by Kinder chocolate – a brand which makes the extremely popular children's 'Kinder Surprise' chocolate egg. The Kinder Surprise Egg, in terms of marketing to children, is quite ingenious. Young children love surprises and they love toys. The people at Kinder managed to link the intense feelings of anticipation and pleasure with chocolate in one easy hit. This kind 'er' direct advertising aimed at children is bad enough, but not only do mass-market chocolate companies use 'fun' and 'happiness' as an emotional pull to lure children in *and* put toys in chocolate eggs, they also deliberately place their products at the height of the average ten-year-old, *and* link chocolate to feel-good films and Disney characters, *and* make sure their bars are on sale in all major children's theme parks, *and*, *and*, *and* … Be under no illusion that whenever you see chocolate, crisp, sweet or fast-food companies raising money to promote 'Books for Schools' or 'Get Active' or such like, that they are doing your kids a favour, the main reason why chocolate companies sponsor schools is:

THEY WANT THEM AS LIFELONG CUSTOMERS!

To achieve this not only will they have posters up in schools and sometimes provide 'free' football strips for the kids with their product plastered all over it (how kind!), but also they often arrange 'exclusive contacts' to put chocolate vending machines in the schools. That way the good feeling of 'having a break' from class gets linked to a chocolate bar. This message is then reinforced as the children go through life with several Derren Brown moments, such as 'Have A Break, Have A Kit Kat', and in no time at all a strong relationship with the product has been established.

WHAT A BUNCH OF WONKERS!

There are even supervised school trips to places such as Cadbury World and Chocolate World. I wish I was kidding, but we actually pay for children to get 'educated' about the history of chocolate at this modern-day Willy Wonka fantasy land. This would be fine as the history of anything can be quite educational, but what we are actually paying for is Cadbury's advertising and emotional hook. The whole tour is one huge marketing ploy aimed at children. As

soon as you enter the make-believe chocolate world everyone is
given a couple of 'free' Cadbury chocolate bars and halfway round
you get another two. On top of that there are plenty of 'free'
chocolate 'shots' throughout the journey. As you continue along
the 2–3 hour tour, advert after advert is being beamed into your
conscious and subconscious mind – there is even an 'advert' stop.
This is a place where you can sit and view on large screen, with
superb sound effects, the many Cadbury ads that have been shown
throughout the decades. One ad which particularly caught my
attention was an old Cadbury's Buttons ad. The picture showed a
young mother feeding a child, probably less than one-year old, a
Button. Such is the power of conditioning, this may seem perfectly
OK in your eyes, but by the time you reach the end of this book
you will see just how outrageous it is. The Cadbury World tour also
has a kiddie's ride taking you on a playful journey through
'Cadabra' – a chocolate wonderland – in a 'beanmobile'. On this
journey there is an automatic photomaker (similar to the rides at
Alton Towers) on which, as you stare at the camera, a caption
reads, instead of 'Say Cheese', 'More Chocolate Please'.

The tour is littered with mind-control Derren Brown moments
like this and it naturally ends with you arriving at the largest
Cadbury chocolate shop in the world! Cadbury World estimated it
would have 250,000 visitors during the first 12 months from
opening in August 1991 – the actual figure was 400,000! That's
nearly half a million people in a country of only 60 million.
Chocolate World in the US saw a massive 2 million visitors in 1996
with each child receiving at least one free bar of chocolate on their
tour. As you now know, it's all about the lifetime value of the
customer and the Willy Wonka world of recruiting new punters
remains the same as it ever was – get them when they're young.

IT'S GOOD TO CALL ... EVEN BETTER TO TEXT!

The biggest threat to this 'get them when they're young' policy has been the unprecedented increase in children using mobile phones. Teenagers now spend a whopping £100,000 a day on text messages and, because they only have a certain amount of pocket money, 'top-up cards' are often gaining preference over chocolate bars. However, the sinister world of chocolate is not about to let that get in its way and is now joining in the text revolution as a means of helping recruit new customers. Cadbury launched a Text 'n' Win campaign, in which children who bought Crunchie, Caramel, Dairy Milk or Fuse bars were invited to text in order to win prizes of up to £5,000. The mobile marketing company Flytxt, who carried out the campaign for Cadbury, were happy to boast: 'The products became the talk of the playground' and they were happy to announce that it produced 'five million participations'.

The chief executive of Cadbury Schweppes, John Sunderland said, 'It gave sales a big lift at a time when the UK confectionery market was pretty flat.' In fact, the campaign was so successful that Cadbury followed up with another texting campaign during the Commonwealth games (and there's me thinking gambling for children was illegal!)

CHOCOLATES R US

Chocolate placement aimed at children couldn't be more obvious than at 'Toys R Us'. Now I thought 'Toys R Us' were simply a toy store. My wild – stab in the dark – suspicions were due to the fact the stores called *Toys R Us*. However, the first thing children see when they enter the warehouse of fun is – chocolate! Not just little bars, no – huge bucket loads of the stuff. Just like a KFC family meal, you can now have your chocolate by the bucket load. The first bucket I saw was for Smarties which had the strap line, 'A Riot

Full of Fun' down its side. How on earth can a load of sugar, fat and powder in an artificially coloured case be a 'riot of fun'? Riot, yes – after all, get a load of kids 'sugared up' and that's precisely what you have on your hands – but fun, no. I then saw mini-buckets of virtually all the most common chocolates, once again conveniently placed at 'child height'.

ADVERTISING DOESN'T EFFECT ME

You may feel that all the advertising, brainwashing, conditioning, trips around Chocolate World and text campaigns have got nothing to do with why *you* eat chocolate. You may simply believe that the only reason you eat it is because it's *sooooooo* blooming lovely. You may also feel that it is fair game for Cadbury and the rest of the chocolate gang to aim their adverts at children. You may strongly think: 'We're not talking cigarettes here Jason, it's only a bit of chocolate.' If that's the case, I shouldn't think you're on your own there; after all, it takes a very open mind to be alive to the possibility that we could have been manipulated on a mental and physical level to this extent, to the possibility that mass-market chocolate could in any way be as harmful for us as cigarettes. However, for you to truly break free you must at least be open to the possibility that conditioning has played a massive part in your apparent decision to buy chocolate. After all, you don't see the average badger yelping for a Yorkie, no matter what time of the month it is, nor what mood it's in!

There is, of course, more to it than just mental conditioning, and one thing I cannot argue with is that like most people reading this book you will firmly believe that you love the taste of the stuff and that life without feeling a cold piece of chocolate melting on your tongue simply would 'not be worth living'. However, please expand your mind as we well and truly strip away this layer by …

4
Licking The Taste!

I mentioned at the start that in order to break free from chocolate you will need an *extremely* open mind. Well, if you can I need you to open your mind even wider for this next revelation – CHOCOLATE TASTES DISGUSTING! Now hang on, before you throw the book in the bin, thinking I'm a few Cadbury's Buttons short of a full jacket, please hear me out. I'm not saying for one second that you don't like the taste of your favourite brand of chocolate, because clearly you do, but what I am saying is that chocolate, in its *unsweetened* state is about as appealing on the taste front as a clip around the ear with a wet kipper. Actually, it's much worse than that. I don't know if you've ever had the misfortune to taste unsweetened cocoa, but trust me it's just not worth it! While researching for this book I made the somewhat catastrophic mistake of getting Cadbury to send me some unsweetened cocoa beans. I decided to conduct my own taste survey amongst my friends – well, when I say friends, after my little experiment they may be ex-friends! I managed to convince 20 people, many of whom describe themselves as 'chocolate lovers', to try these not-so-tasty treats. The results were pretty conclusive – 95% of the people surveyed spat out the bean and were nearly physically sick. There was only one person who managed to eat and swallow it, but even then she thought it tasted like crap.

If you're in any doubt at all and think I may be exaggerating for effect, please pop along to Cadbury World and ask them if you can taste one of their 'unsweetened' cocoa beans (oh, and don't forget your bucket!). Or if you can't make it there, go on the hunt for some high-percentage cocoa chocolate. Now when I say high percentage, I'm not talking 70% dark chocolate bars – these have still been heavily sweetened with sugar – no, I'm talking 95–99% chocolate solids (once again make sure there's a toilet nearby). This is because, as I will continue to say, chocolate in its unsweetened state is revolting. Actually, revolting is being rather nice! As I write this chapter I've just had another unsweetened cocoa bean to fully associate with what I'm trying to get across – and what I have just tasted is almost indescribable and in my mind I've only ever tasted one other thing which is worse. Have you ever woken up from a party and felt so thirsty that you reached for the nearest can of whatever to quench your thirst, only to discover (too late) it contained cigarette ash? Well, that's what we're talking about here!

The main ingredient which causes the foul taste is a naturally occurring powerful heart stimulant called theobromine. Theobromine is incredibly bitter and the darker the chocolate, the more 'real chocolate' it contains and the *worse* it tastes. Our taste buds are designed to warn us of poisons – if something tastes bitter it usually means that nature never intended us to eat it. Chocolate has always tasted as bitter as a winter's night in Scotland and has always been sweetened to make it palatable. When the Aztec civilizations of Central America first started using chocolate a couple of thousand years ago (depending on what you read!) it was nothing like the chocolate we get today. Firstly, they only drank it, the chocolate 'bar' only came in around 1847 when Joseph Fry (as in Fry's Chocolate) discovered that by adding chocolate liquor and sugar to cocoa butter he could produce a solid chocolate. And the drinking chocolate they had then was certainly a few chemicals and spoonfuls of sugar short of the hot cocoa your parents used to tuck you up in bed with, that's for sure. Back then the drink was extremely bitter and spicy, thickened with maize and flavoured with vanilla, ginger and even chilli and turmeric (yum, yum!). But the Aztecs didn't go to all this trouble because they thought drinking it helped with the stresses and strains of life or because they thought it was something they could 'have in-between meals without ruining their appetite' or because they thought it tasted good! No, they only started drinking it because they thought they were honouring their principle God, Quetzalcoatl-Tlahuizcalpanticutli (the God of light), in much the same way some Christians take bread and wine at communion, the Aztecs honestly thought the pods were gifts from God, hence their naming the cocoa the 'food of the Gods'. The name of the tree from which the beans come from is *Theobroma cacao*, which literally translates as 'god food'.

MONEY TO BURN

This belief led to the beans being held in very high esteem, so much so that in the land of the Aztecs, the beans were more precious than gold. Cocoa beans were literally their currency and were exchanged for many goods and services. But because the beans were not only as good as money, but in those days *were* money, only the very wealthiest of people could roast and drink them. In fact, it was only those who literally had 'money to burn' who ever got to taste drinking chocolate (and that's where the saying comes from!).

For the Aztecs, drinking chocolate was never about 'Having A Break' and it certainly wasn't about the taste – it was about honouring their God, ceremonial occasions, religious beliefs and showing great wealth. It seems funny that in those days they made the 'sacrifice' of drinking this muck in order to honour their God and show off – now we have a nation that feels that they would be making a sacrifice by *not* having it. That's because what we have today and what they had then are not remotely the same thing. But if you still feel that back then it could have been all about the taste, then this should seal it. In Aztecs times, priests would mix cocoa with the blood of human sacrifices and force their victims to drink it. Even now there are Italian villagers who make a concoction called 'sanguinaccio' which is a wonderful dish of stewed pig's blood, numerous other ingredients and, of course, some grated black chocolate ('see the face you love, and throw up' springs to mind).

While we are talking about the taste of chocolate, it's worth knowing that the Aztecs 'special drink' was called 'chocolatl' – literally meaning 'bitter water'. Just to make this point crystal clear, the only reason they drank this incredibly bitter concoction was because they strongly believed it brought universal wisdom and knowledge which continued into the afterlife. It certainly wasn't because of the taste! (Glad that's now clear.) But even when the chocolate 'bar' was eventually born, and the vast majority of people had stopped mixing blood with their cocoa (good move!), it still needed heavily sweetening to gain universal appeal.

MANIPULATING YOUR TASTE BUDS

There are some people who love the taste of very dark chocolate and there are a few weird people who even like the unsweetened cocoa bean. But then let's not forget, there are some people who say they like the *taste* of cigarettes and yet they never eat them and there is even a group of people in the world who drink their own urine. However, just because this floats the boat for a few people, I don't believe this shows that it is a genuinely lovely taste and something we should all be doing!

Our taste buds, just like our minds, can easily be moulded and conditioned. As part of our natural survival mechanism, our taste buds are designed to adapt to *any* foods we are presented with on a regular basis. This is why, just like our minds, they can easily be fooled. For example, when you had your first alcoholic drink, did you jump for joy exclaiming, 'Where have you been all my life?' I don't think so! The vast majority of children/teenagers simply think, 'What the hell is this rubbish, give me an orange juice.' Yet, as we persevered with the taste of a particular brand we gradually acquired a liking for it. But even then, we're not actually enjoying the taste of the alcohol itself. Neat alcohol not only feels like you've just set fire to your mouth, but it can kill you instantly! What you enjoy is a mixture of added flavours and chemicals which are there to try and mask the taste of alcohol. Now don't panic, this book isn't about getting rid of alcohol (phew!), I just wanted to point out that cocoa is similar in terms of taste. In its neat form its taste is awful so it needs to be covered up, otherwise there would be no GODS and no 'love' of chocolate. In the case of alcohol we have products such as alcopops. One of the reasons for their success is because they don't taste of alcohol at all; instead they have been designed to taste like orange, lemon, blackberry, etc, so slowly but surely manipulating the taste buds.

The difference with alcohol and chocolate is that you don't have your first shot of alcohol when you are still in a buggy! This is why the alcohol companies have to work harder initially to manipulate our minds, and then do the same with our taste buds as most have been developed by the time we have our first hit. But with chocolate it's a whole different kettle of creme eggs. It seems perfectly normal and natural to mix in some chocolate powder with a baby's milk before they've even learnt to pronounce 'Ovaltine', let alone make a conscious decision to make some for themselves. If you were fed 'neat' cocoa as a child you would spit it out since your body's natural defence mechanism would kick in and scream, 'This is a type of poison – stop doing it.' If you're in any doubt, give your dog high-percentage cocoa-rich chocolates, second thoughts don't as you would run a considerable risk of killing them – yes, killing them! The high concentrations of theobromine found in dark chocolate can easily send the heart of your dog racing so fast that it has an attack. Humans are more robust when it comes to this heart stimulant, but the natural tendency to spit out neat cocoa should still tell us that it is not good for us. However, if all you were presented with on a regular basis was neat cocoa powder, your body *would* eventually adapt and you *would* end up acquiring a taste for the 'hard stuff' of the chocolate world. This is why people can end up believing they like the taste of cigarettes – proof in itself that our amazing survival mechanisms and taste buds can adjust to just about anything (except Brussels sprouts – I don't think they fall into this category!)

So considering that the chocolate we were presented with as kids had already been 'alcopop-ed' as it were, with sugar,chemicals and artificial flavourings, and since we were given these bars/boxs/slabs by way of a 'reward' at times when we were feeling good anyway, is it any wonder that the vast majority of people acquire a relationship *and* taste for the stuff?

Because our taste buds are conditioned to what *we* are presented with over and over and over again, the relationship built up with chocolate will depend on the culture in which you are brought up. The British tend to like the caramelized flavour of Cadbury's, the Swiss prefer milkier chocolate such as Lindt and Toblerone, the Italians prefer the darker bitter creamier chocolate such as Baci and the US like Hershey chocolate – a brand that just doesn't cut the nougat overseas with a taste that's been described as 'burned leaves and toasted rubber'. In fact, to the pretentious chocolate connoisseurs, Hershey chocolate is considered 'offensive' if not completely 'inedible'. Hans Schu, a Swiss national, goes one further by saying, 'Milton Hershey completely ruined the American palate with his sour, gritty chocolate … he had no idea what he was doing. Who in their right mind would set out to produce such a sour chocolate?' A friend of mine who travels to the States on a regular basis said that 'Hershey chocolate tastes like sick.' However, to the chocolate-loving people in the US, Hershey chocolate tastes blooming lovely, thank you very much. It's only the European chocolate 'connoisseurs' who profess that it doesn't taste as chocolate should – but how should chocolate taste? Well, in reality no one knows.

Unlike other 'foods', chocolate doesn't have an official 'chocolate taste'. Strawberry is strawberry, orange is orange, and lemon is lemon no matter where you go in the world, but chocolate is always a little different. This is because each variety of cocoa bean produces its own unique perfume and each results in a different chocolate taste. Also, each different method, different milk and different chemical used in the making of chocolate produces different flavours. So, it is not the taste of 'chocolate' you love, as all chocolate tastes different, it is the taste of the variety *you* are used to, the variety that was fed to *you* before your taste buds had a personality of their own. And the chances are, unless you are one of the rare few who like only 99% cocoa solid chocolate (which I doubt, as you wouldn't be 'hooked' so you wouldn't even be reading this book), then you don't actually like the taste of chocolate at all. What you have been *conditioned* to like is some bitter tasting powder that's been covered and processed with all kinds of addictive rubbish to make it taste sweet and creamy.

'BUT JASON – EVERYONE KNOWS IT'S BETTER THAN SEX'

Even though the mass-market sweetened, chemically-driven chocolates, taste much, much better than high-percentage cocoa solids, I would still argue that the whole 'delicious … unique …

orgasmic' taste thing is one massive exaggerated story. Think about it – we all have stories where we have exaggerated them slightly to give it a little more spark. Now sometimes we say the same story so often that in the end even we end up believing it. Is it possible that exactly the same thing could have happened with the 'taste' and 'feelings' of chocolate? Is it possible that all this 'Oh, the way it melts in your mouth' or 'It's simply orgasmic, better than sex' is in reality a load of old tosh?

Like so many things in life, the *idea* of having it is much better than the reality and what we must realize is that the *idea* of the fabulous taste of chocolate is constantly being perpetuated by the media, advertising, the GODS and, funny enough, by ourselves! Haven't you been out for a meal and tried to sell the *idea* of a chocolate dessert to others so you were not alone in your drug-food moment. And didn't you exaggerate it, oh so slightly?

You know, 'Go on, how about some delicious, ice-cool chocolate ice-cream?' or 'They do a devilishly gorgeous full chocolate gateau – go on, you only live once.' In truth, once the GODS have got us, they might as well save their money on advertising – we end up doing it for them for free! But why? What is *sooooooo* special about the taste? Show me one person who actually puts a piece of chocolate into their mouth *slowly*, lets it melt *slowly*, and *slowly* savours the flavours, and I'll drink some of that sanguinaccio! The truth is we're on to the next chocolate or bite of bar before the first has had a chance to hit the sides. All this stuff *we* expound – 'It's simply heaven', 'It's better than sex' – in truth (excuse my French), it's all bollocks, isn't it? It's stuff we've said and heard said over the years and it's a neat way, if we're honest (?), of helping to justify our intake.

Let's look at the Flake ad again. There she is, a beautiful, *slim* woman, not a care in the world, in a bathroom that's bigger than my flat. She is orally, seductively having a Flake in the bath. Impression – it's better than sex! Have you ever actually tried eating a Flake in the bath? You get bits stuck on the roof of your mouth, bits in the bath and you never really know what to do with those bits left in the wrapper. You make a sort of funnel with the wrapper, place one end in your mouth and turn yourself into a human chute, praying you don't get it everywhere. You then say, 'Oh, I wish I hadn't had that' – funny how you don't see this on the Flake ad, isn't it? Britney Spears was once quoted as saying, 'Chocolate for me is just like an orgasm' (she needs to get out more!). Having a bar of chocolate is *not* better than sex, no matter how often people say it. However, if you actually do believe that, then instead of eating more, trying to attain that pleasure, may I make a suggestion – CHANGE YOUR PARTNER! (or buy some chocolate love toys.)

DAYLIGHT SNOBBERY

The taste thing has, like with wine, got completely out of hand. Now there are even professional chocolate tasters and official chocolate connoisseurs – once again the word 'bollocks' springs to mind. At Mars' chocolate-making plant in the US, a panel of professional chocolate tasters meet every day to taste the goods. You may think that this sounds like the best job in the world, but like wine tasters, they're not allowed to swallow, and the chocolate they taste hasn't even been sweetened. So if you think about the roasted cocoa beans from Cadbury and my friends wanting to be sick, all of a sudden the job doesn't sound so dreamy.

But it is the pretentious so-called connoisseurs of chocolate who really expose this taste sensation nonsense for what it is. Just like their 'look at me, I've got an education' wine-tasting cousins, these choco-connoisseurs come out with the biggest load of bullshit in order to make themselves sound important. If you think wine tasters sound pathetic as they drink some gone-off fruit and fermented vegetation while proclaiming to the world that it has a good nose, full body and is 'somewhat mysterious' before spitting it into a bucket, that is nothing compared to the chocolate gang. There they are at the annual chocolate tasting convention (yes, there is such a thing) putting pieces of chocolate on their tongues, letting it melt slightly, then spitting it out – while proclaiming, no doubt, that it has a 'distinctive West African gusto', a '1945 Swiss feel about it' and, once again, it probably is 'somewhat mysterious'. The mystery is how these people get the vote! Do you think they've been saying this sort of stuff for so long that they now believe what they're saying?

CHOCOLATE THERAPY

If you think that's barking, then what do you think of this next chap? His name is Murray Langham, author of the book *Chocolate Therapy: Unwrap the Secrets of Your Inner Self*. I was once on a radio programme with this guy when he was launching his book in the UK – he was on the phone from the States and I was in a BBC studio here in England. I don't want to mock but 'HELLO, IS THERE ANYBODY HOME?' He claims that depending on the taste and shape of the chocolate you like, it not only determines part of your future but also tells you the kind of person you are. For example, if you like the taste of chocolate, 'you are part of the advancement of the human race, looking to the future. You're a pro-active person who respects other people's points of view …' and so it goes on. He then says that if you don't like chocolate then '… perhaps you need to see a chocolate therapist.' Now I realize that most people haven't advanced to this level of far-out theory to sell the idea of chocolate to themselves and others, but you may not be lagging that far behind!

CONFECTIONERY

The fact is, you are *not* addicted because of the taste. You have certainly acquired a taste for it, there's no question of that, and, yes, possibly you do now love the flavour of your favourite 'brand' of chocolate. But what must be clear is that is not *why* you find it hard to stop eating it. I love freshly picked strawberries. I love the texture, the look, the taste, the way a cool strawberry on a hot summer's day feels in the mouth. I love the way that once in the mouth it begins to soften and melt, the flavours slowly trickling down my throat. I love all of that, but after I've had one I don't have to 'hammer the rest home' until I feel sick; I don't have to try and sell them to myself with provocative words or get people to 'join me' without feeling guilty. And if they were making me fat, ill, miserable and spotty I certainly wouldn't have to buy a book on how to stop eating them! I don't mean to shout but this point must be clear before we move on:

YOU ARE NOT ADDICTED BECAUSE OF THE TASTE!

You need to understand the reason for the 'hook' isn't simply down to a very clever manipulating and manufactured taste, but the whole brainwashing package. And it's the brainwashing package that needs looking at most of all. Taste clearly *does* come into it, I'm not saying for one second it doesn't, and like I say you have indeed acquired more than a simple taste that you possibly now like very much, but you need to realize even the taste is a con. Not only are there professionals who are paid massive amounts of money to trick your taste buds and who can literally make anything taste of anything. Taste technology is now so advanced that they can make an artificial taste of vanilla if they so wish. Every aspect of the 'taste sensation' has been cleverly designed to trick you and, more importantly, to make sure that you come back for more. You need to realize that the chemicals and other apparent 'foods' they use to cover up the foul taste of cocoa also create part of the mental hook. The reason? Some are highly addictive!

We have seen already that there are many layers to this chocolate wolf – advertising, conditioning, brainwashing and taste. But each segment has its own layer and each one needs stripping fully before you can even begin to make the mental shift to freedom. Remember, I don't expect you to get rid of chocolate yet, please tuck in if you want to throughout your reading of this book. We need to remove *every* layer and *then* give you the mental guidance before you can make the jump (glad that's clear!).

On the taste front, we now know that neat cocoa tastes awful. In order to make it taste good the GODS have had to apply several different layers in order to make it edible and appealing for the mass market. The taste of cocoa is bitter, so therefore easily *resistible*. To help make it apparently 'irresistible', combinations of different confectioneries are made. It's worth knowing that the word 'confection' originally referred to a 'medicine' made palatable with the addition of spices and sugar, hence, in my book – *con*fection. Yes, even back in the 18th century, long before the chocolate bar was upon us and long before the GODS were doing the manipulating, doctors, along with priests, were preaching the 'benefits' of the bitter chocolate brew and were calling it a medicine. And how do we get the medicine to go down? A spoonful of sugar, of course! Now call me Mr Cynical, but it comes as no great surprise to me that doctors and priests were celebrating the virtues of this confection. Yep, you guessed it: the main manufacturers of chocolate brew were … priests and doctors! The GODS, of course, have gone a lot further than this with the addition of chemicals and all kinds of other 'goodies'. However, there is one thing which hasn't changed since the birth of the chocolate bar. There are a few substances in mass-market chocolate which hold your taste buds hostage, but make no mistake, none have the same power as this next layer. Yes, willpower doesn't stand a chance, as your taste buds cry …

5

Sweet, Sweet Surrender

It has been described as, 'Pure, White and Deadly', 'The Cocaine of the Food World' and is known to be responsible for more cases of obesity and diabetes than any other single 'food' product on the planet – yes, we're talking sugar. Not just any old sugar you understand, we're talking pure white refined sugar. Make no mistake, without the addition of this empty drug food the chances are you wouldn't even be reading this book. This is the stuff which covers the bitter taste of cocoa and at the same time turns an otherwise *fairly* innocent bean into a very, very addictive substance.

SIMPLE UNNATURAL GLUCOSE, ADDICTIVE AND REFINED

William Duffy was one of the first to warn of the dangers and addictive nature of this substance in his excellent book *Sugar Blues*. Since then there have been many more books warning of the dangers of this apparent 'sweet and innocent' food, and if there's one ingredient in chocolate which I feel more passionate about than any other it is white refined sugar. If you get nothing else from this book, I truly hope that you leave it understanding the full implications of putting white refined sugar into your bloodstream on a regular basis.

The chocolate industry is fully aware of the horrific consequences which can easily come about as a direct result of refined sugar consumption/addiction – consequences which go way, way beyond losing the odd tooth or twenty. Yet despite knowing this, it doesn't stop them lacing their 'aimed-at-children' products with tonnes of the white stuff. As a group, chocolate companies are one of the largest buyers of sugar in the world and they are more than aware of its addictive nature. According to the official BBC website,

'All modern commercial chocolate products contain *substantial* amounts of sugar, a fact which may partly explain chocolate's supposed addictive properties.'

The BBC have it right on the Cadbury button. Cadbury alone get through a massive 150 tonnes of sugar EVERY DAY! That's a whopping 540,000 tonnes of white refined sugar entering just the Cadbury UK chocolate chain every year. With Cadbury chocolate plants in much of the Commonwealth, the collective Cadbury sugar consumption must easily reach millions of tonnes every year. But this enormous figure no doubt pales into insignificance compared to what the Mars boys and girls must get through. I say 'no doubt' because trying to get any information from Mars (or Master Foods, as they're known) is harder than getting close to an elephant's scrotum. One thing is sure, though: with an average mass-market chocolate bar containing a massive 40% sugar, you can be George Bernard Shaw that the annual amount if piled high would probably reach the planet Mars itself. And it is not just Master Foods – the entire chocolate industry plays down the amount of sugar in their products and they have every reason to. They will also use any other word they possibly can on their labels instead of actually saying 'sugar'. Here's what the label says on a Mars Bar wrapper in 2003:

Milk chocolate with soft nougat (33%) and caramel centre (27%)

Sounds all jolly good – 'soft nougat' and a 'caramel centre'. But what the hell is nougat? Nougat is nothing more than eggs, air and SUGAR! When you see a list of ingredients on a food wrapper you probably know they start with the highest percentage ingredient. What are the first two ingredients on a Mars Bar? SUGAR and GLUCOSE SYRUP (more commonly known as SUGAR!). Renaming it 'nougat' or 'syrup' doesn't make it better. You can be almost certain that virtually everything with chocolate written on it is loaded with white refined sugar. Chocolate breakfast cereal is 39% sugar and plain chocolate biscuits are 33% sugar – that's just the added sugar, and doesn't even take into account the biscuit and refined cereal itself which will also turn into sugar once in the bloodstream. If you combined the two you will see that it is virtually all sugar!

DOING A 'SUNNY D'

The chocolate industry is very clever at doing what I call a 'Sunny D' when it comes to advertising. That is, they don't actually lie in their ads, but they are sometimes unbelievably economical with the truth and incredibly misleading. Sunny D ran a radio ad in the summer of 2003 which went something like this.

> 'Which contains less sugar, a bowl of spinach or a glass of new sugar-free Sunny D? Yes, the answer is a glass of new sugar-free Sunny D.'

and then they continued to repeat this point by saying,

> 'That's right; a bowl of spinach actually contains MORE sugar than a glass of new sugar-free Sunny Delight.'

Now the statement happens to be true, but how misleading can you get? Sugar-free Sunny D does indeed have less sugar than spinach, but the small amount of natural sugar in spinach is incredibly good for you. On top of that, they fail to mention in their ad that new sugar-free Sunny D contains artificial sweeteners sweeteners that have been linked to many health problems, including brain tumours!

Just so you know why I'm so against sugar, let me explain exactly what happens on a mental and physical level when you eat or drink it and then precisely what the potential long and short-term health risks are.

GOOD LOOKING, SO REFINED – LIKE TO KNOW WHAT IT'S DOING TO YOUR MIND?

What harm can a little refining do? Just the word 'refining' gives the impression that something has been in some way improved upon. However, not only does refining sugar not improve the original sugar cane or beet, but it transforms it into a very dangerous drug-like substance. When sugar cane is 'refined', *all* the vitamins are destroyed. What difference can a few vitamins make? Well, in the 17th and 18th centuries many people lost their lives in a very short space of time due to a lack of a few vitamins, the most famous being vitamin C. Scurvy wiped out over 4,000 mariners in about two years. In the end the 'cure' was a simple lemon or orange, each packed with natural sugars, fats, vitamins, minerals, water and amino acids – the six essential human needs. When sugar is 'refined' the natural balance of the food is upset. Every food that nature produces for human consumption is as carefully constructed as the human body itself. Each and every molecule is designed to work synergistically to maintain and run the body as efficiently as possible. You cannot interfere with the fine mechanics of nature's food and expect everything to be OK. If you stripped away a number of components from motor oil your car wouldn't run the same way and exactly the same applies to nature's food and your body. Without the vitamins, minerals and fibres, not only does your body experience 'lack' and so feel 'empty', it also sends sugar into the bloodstream far too rapidly.

White refined sugar is stripped to such a degree that it goes more or less straight through the stomach and enters the bloodstream *instantly*. This was not what nature had in mind! Food is meant to be digested in the stomach before being passed on to the intestines where the energy and nutrients can be *slowly* absorbed. But as all the vitamins, minerals and fibres have been destroyed (sorry, I mean refined!) the body sees no reason to go through this process. The instant rush of glucose (sugar) you get when you eat white refined sugar causes your blood sugar levels to rocket, thus causing a massive imbalance in the blood. This imbalance must be quickly rectified otherwise you will die (pretty important then!). The body has no alternative but to call on the pancreas to produce some of the 'fat-producing' hormone insulin. Let me repeat that as many reading this book will be doing so with their weight in mind – the 'FAT-PRODUCING' HORMONE insulin. This is the stuff that takes excess calories and literally pushes them into fat cells. It's worth knowing that the 'rush' you feel when you eat a mass-market chocolate bar or drink a sugar-infested 'soft' drink (or both combined!) is not due to natural energy-boosting properties of the 'food' or drink itself, but is mainly down to insulin shooting through your bloodstream trying to burn off the excess sugar. Once the insulin has burnt the excess glucose from the bloodstream – removing the *immediate* danger – it then has the job of getting rid of it. It does this by transporting some of the excess sugar to the liver and muscles for 'short-term' energy use, the rest is transported to your 'FAT CELLS'. Because the pancreas had no alternative but to *over*-secrete insulin, the excess sugar in the bloodstream was burnt very rapidly. This often causes you to have hypoglycaemia, better known as *low* blood sugar. I'm going to repeat this as it is very important and not something that most people realize (since the opposite *appears real*):

SUGAR CAUSES ... *LOW* BLOOD SUGAR!

Yes, bizarre as that may sound, white refined sugar causes *low* blood sugar. And when you feel the effects of low blood sugar what do you look for? Yep – more of the same to give you a 'lift'. How brilliant is that for the GODS? After all, surely the main problem with being in the food industry is that once people have eaten your product you have satisfied their hunger and so, in theory, you have to wait until they're hungry again before you can sell them more food. Unless, of course, you found a way to create 'false hungers'. And unless you found a way of making people feel hungrier more often than they otherwise would. A way of *creating* empty insecure feelings of *dissatisfaction* in the bloodstream – a dissatisfied feeling which only appears to be satisfied by more of the same. Imagine how clever that would be? Imagine if you could fool people into believing they were getting *satisfied* with the very substances which were causing them to feel *dissatisfied?* Well, there really is no need to imagine, as this is precisely what the mass-market chocolate industry have been doing for years and it is one of the main reasons why many people are well and truly 'hooked' on the stuff. By lacing their products with massive amounts of white refined sugar and other addictive chemicals, they know this will cause a rapid rise in blood-sugar levels, which in turn forces the body to over-secrete insulin, which then burns off the excess sugar and thus, in a much shorter time than usual, causes blood sugar to fall and create a feeling of dissatisfaction. Because the blood-sugar levels are now lower than normal, *caused* by the sugar and additives in the last dose, nothing else will seem to hit the mark other than some more of the same. This is why when you feel the empty insecure feelings of low-blood sugar, you don't crave a piece of fish!

JUST THE ONE

The GODS also know that it is only when your sugar levels begin to stabilize that you can feel satisfied, so the minute you eat a piece of mass-market chocolate it will immediately trigger a release of insulin in your bloodstream and so you will *instantly* feel hungrier than you did a second earlier. This creates an instant 'false hunger' and is one of the reasons why you may well have thought, 'Oh, just the one', but ended up having two, three or, as likely as not, devouring the whole box. This factor, cleverly combined with the naturally occurring addictive stimulant theobromine (found in cocoa), the added caffeine, milk and an array of other ingredients worthy of any chemical convention, leaves you with the mother of all battles – a battle which you seemingly can never win! You either use your willpower to stop yourself having more while at the same time feeling mentally deprived, or you tuck in, devour the lot and feel like crap – what a choice! It's worth knowing that this mental tug-of-war is no accident and has nothing to do with your personality. The mass-market chocolate companies work hard to make certain they produce an empty 'food' specifically designed to leave you dissatisfied and to keep you coming back for more. They even have the front to tell us this (and we seem not to notice). Remember this?

'A Chocolate Bar You Can Eat In-Between Meals Without Ruining Your Appetite'

I thought the whole point of eating *was* to ruin your appetite, to satisfy your hunger. They are blatantly telling us that this 'food' is something you can eat in-between meals without ruining your hunger. In that case it should be pretty obvious that it's not real food. Imagine saying to a squirrel, 'Here's a nut you can eat in-between nuts without ruining your nutty appetite' – how nuts would that be? Yet here we are, perhaps the most intelligent species on the planet, falling for this nonsense. What they are really saying is, 'Here's a chocolate bar which will take the edge off of your "false sugar" hunger, but will not interfere with your *genuine* appetite and need for "live" nutrients.'

'I'll buy a huge piece of meat, cook it up for dinner, and then right before it's done, I'll break down and have what I wanted for dinner in the first place – bread and jam … all I ever really want is SUGAR.' [my emphasis]

Andy Warhol, *New York Magazine*, March 31, 1975

Like any good drug company, the chocolate industry lace their wares with addictive substances and empty nutrients with the sole objective of leaving you feeling empty and wanting more. One crisp manufacturer even boasts that 'Once You Pop You Cannot Stop', and as you will certainly now realize that the same applies when you 'dip' into a box of mass-market, high-fat and sugar, chemically-laced chocolates. Interestingly, the same urge to have more and more does *not* usually occur with 99% cocoa chocolate. This kind of chocolate does *not* raise sugar levels rapidly, does *not* cause your system to over-secrete insulin and does not push fats into your arteries (more on that later). However, 99% cocoa chocolate *does* still have the stimulants theobromine and caffeine, and in *much* higher quantities than is found in mass-market chocolate. But the awful bitter taste is usually enough to override any possible addiction – in fact, it's usually enough to override any desire to eat the stuff at all. The truth is, when it comes to chocolate, the over-secretion of insulin *only* occurs with the mass-market stuff that has been heavily laced with white refined sugar and chemicals. This is why, in the words of Joel Glenn Brenner, the author of the magnificent book, *The Chocolate Wars*:

'… each swallow of M&Ms leaves you with an insidious craving.'

According to Brenner's book, Allan Gibbons of Mars echoes this sentiment by explaining:

'We test people in our offices. We'd give them a bowl of M&Ms every day, about a pound, I guess. And they'd have them on their desks and just be grazing away. We'd gauge how much they liked the product by how much they physically ate.'

So, you see, it really is no accident that chocolate often leaves you with an almost uncontrollable desire for more and more. Clearly there is eventually a cut-off point when your body gives the signal of 'enough is enough', usually by telling you that unless you stop you're going to throw up, or when your brain kicks in and says, 'Stop I don't want to get fat!' The body then goes about its business of trying to deal with the rubbish. Once again the excess sugar is transported to the liver, muscles and fat cells, and once again the sugar levels *drop* earlier than normal causing a feeling of dissatisfaction and an empty insecure feeling in the bloodstream. These feelings are virtually identical to other normal dissatisfied feelings in life, such as stress, boredom, anxiety and general feelings of insecurity. The chocolate and sweet industries play on this by giving the *false* impression in their £1m marketing campaigns that your genuine feelings of emptiness can be filled with their 'foods' and 'drinks'. The problem is … their ads *do* work. But why? Because, when you eat sugar-loaded products such as mass-market chocolate, the empty insecure feelings of low blood sugar or 'false hunger' are *immediately* lifted and so seem to confirm what the ads are saying. This not only makes people believe that *genuine* emotions can indeed be lessened with high sugar products such as chocolate, but it also adds to the illusion of 'pleasure you can't measure'.

PLEASURE YOU *CAN* MEASURE!

Well, unluckily for the GODS, the pleasure *can* now be measured and like the whole concept of mass-market chocolate, it's shown to be false! The GODS are cleverly playing on our natural insecurities, natural hunger feelings and natural pleasures. Eating food and ending a natural hunger is pleasurable, especially with something which tastes sweet. The pleasure, though, is simply the ending of the empty insecure aggravation we know as hunger or the ending of an unnatural 'mental wanting'. Ending any kind of aggravation, whether mental of physical, is pleasurable. All the GODS are doing is to cause us to feel more hunger, or more 'mentally' deprived more often, so creating the illusion that they 'give us' more pleasure more often. But they *are not* giving more pleasure; they are simply creating more aggravations and more false feelings of dissatisfaction.

The 'aggravations' can manifest themselves in all kinds of ways and what I describe as 'withdrawal symptoms' from white refined sugar usually occur within three hours after consuming some. In many cases these come in the shape of headaches, dizziness, sweating, tremors, increased heart rate, depression or, most commonly, slight irritability, anxiety and *hunger*. If at that moment you eat some chocolate loaded with sugar what happens? Yep – the symptoms subside, the aggravation appears to end and you feel *pleasure*. But this kind of pleasure is akin to banging your hand with a mallet simply to get the relief and pleasure of when you finally stop! Who in their right mind would deliberately cause any kind of aggravation with the sole purpose of seeking the pleasure of ending it?

SUGAR ROBS YOU OF YOUR ENERGY

Not only is the mental *and* physical 'pleasure' pretty much an illusion, but so too is the rubbish about sugar giving you energy. Not only has the sugar industry banged on about 'sugar giving you energy' for years, but many chocolate companies even have the audacity to promote their products as 'energy boosting'; once again it's complete bullshit. When you feel 'low blood sugar' your energy levels *drop* and you feel sluggish. What *causes* very low blood sugar? Yep – SUGAR! William Duffy, bestselling author of *Sugar Blues* wrote about sugar:

> 'Here is something more intoxicating than beer or wine and more potent than many drugs and potions then known to man ... it was a brain boggier. It could cause the human body and brain to run the gamut in no time at all from exhaustion to hallucination.'

'Hallucination' is perhaps the best word and it pretty much sums up what most sugar addicts experience. They are all under the hallucination that sugar is an energy-boosting pleasure food. For years it was an established 'fact' that the world was flat and all those who thought otherwise were considered barking mad. The truth is that they weren't mad at all – in reality they were very enlightened. They opened their mind to see beyond the accepted truth. And this is exactly what you need to do to free yourself of sugar-infested mass-market chocolate and, while we're here, any refined sugar-laced 'instant hit' drug food. Sugar only *appears* to give you energy because you feel a slight *lift* from the sluggish feeling of a sugar *low*: A sugar low which was in all likelihood *caused* by your last 'fix' of white refined sugar itself.

This 'sugar merry-go-round' is bad enough in itself and it keeps people enslaved to a drug-like substance. However, the chocolate companies might perhaps be forgiven this if this was the end of the problem. After all, aren't most businesses guilty of attempting to create the illusion that our lives would be in some way empty if we didn't buy their product or service? Isn't this the very essence of business and sales? But we aren't talking about shampoo or soap powder here; we're talking about an *extremely* toxic and addictive substance. We are talking about something which goes *into the bloodstream* of the 'customer' and causes unbelievable disease of the mind and body.

'BUT JASON, IT'S ONLY A BIT OF SUGAR ... ISN'T IT?'

You may well think I'm going a bit over the top about what you might see as 'a bit of sugar', but what I want to make crystal clear is that it isn't *just a bit* of sugar – it is up to 40% worth in just one bar! To your body that is not *just a bit* of sugar. A mere two ounces of white refined sugar entering the bloodstream is enough to cause a *major* upset and imbalance in the fine workings of the human body and mind. I know it may be hard to get your head round the fact that sugar can be as harmful as other white-powder drugs, but we have to remember that it took many, many years before the tobacco companies, governments (and even us), began to entertain the idea that a toxic and highly dangerous poison like nicotine could in anyway be harmful. In fact, a few years ago if anyone dared to suggest that cigarettes were in any way bad for you, they either hugely discredited you and/or sued. Now, of course, matters are very different and there are massive warnings on cigarette packets, and adverts showing people with cancer and warning of the horrific dangers are commonplace. However, the mental and physical illness caused by smoking actually pales into insignificance compared to that of white refined sugar and in the addiction stakes many believe sugar holds the same addictive power as heroin. Yet, despite the overwhelming and obvious evidence linking white refined sugar to a multitude of mental and physical disorders, at this time there are no plans to put any type of warning on the packets containing these highly dangerous white refined granules.

A SPOONFUL OF SUGAR … MAKES THE MEDICINE GO DOWN

Many people have written about sugar, but there are two whose opinions are really worth listening to. In 1956, Surgeon-Captain TL Cleave, MRCP, formerly Director of Medical Research of the Institute of Naval Medicine in the UK went as far as to say, 'the saccharine disease' was the master disease. He explained this 'master disease' incorporated diabetes, coronary disease, varicose veins, *E. coli* infections, obesity, constipation, haemorrhoids, appendicitis, many skin conditions and a list which goes on way beyond what we have room for here. Dr Cleave and his associates also noted what many before and after them have:

> 'There is one common factor in all traditional *healthy* diets: the absence of sugar and all simple carbohydrates.'

That's simple carbohydrates such as white refined sugar and white flour, both of which are to be found in your regular mass-market chocolate muffins, cakes and bars.

In 1929, Dr Frederick Banting, the scientist who discovered insulin, tried to tell the world that his discovery is *not* a cure at all and that the only way to prevent diabetes was to cut down on 'dangerous' sugar bingeing. He went on to state:

> 'In the U.S. the incidence of diabetes has increased proportionately with the per capita consumption of sugar.'

His warning has done nothing to stop this trend. Diabetes has more than tripled since 1958, once again right in line with the consumption of sugar. It is now becoming common to know someone with diabetes, yet a little over 100 years ago only 1% of the Western world had the disease. Not only are more people contracting Type 2 diabetes, but the victims of this are getting younger and younger. There is now a huge increase in teenage Type 2 diabetes, caused, according to the 'Get Active' brigade, by a lack of exercise and not by milky cocoa products containing loads of white refined sugar.

Many people believe what I used to about diabetes: that it is a slightly unfortunate and inconvenient disease to have but, other than having to inject insulin every now and then (if type 1) or having to control your diet a bit (if type 2 – the most common), there isn't a lot more to it. What I didn't know was that people can easily lose their eyesight and limbs because of this disease – a disease for which sugar is *known* to be the number one major cause. I watched an extremely graphic programme about sugar which showed how one lady became blind in her early 30s simply because of her addiction to white refined sugar-laced foods (which obviously included mass-market chocolate). Getting cancer because you smoke is one thing, but not being able to see because of a food which has passed all government checks is nothing short of outrageous. Another image in this programme showed graphic pictures of people with gangrenous arms and legs, prior to having them amputated! So the harmless 'oh, it's only a bit of sugar' granules are *not only* the single number one cause of obesity on the planet but *also* the number one cause of diabetes – a disease which is so horrific that people up and down the country are going blind and having parts of their body removed because of it. It now becomes clear why obesity and diabetes are so tightly linked – sugar is the major cause of both. It is this simple: a sudden surge of simple sugar in the bloodstream creates a response from the pancreas to secrete the fat-producing hormone insulin. Every time this happens the pancreas is overworked, running the huge risk of wearing it out. A worn-out pancreas = diabetes!

Many athletic, slim, sporty people are deluded into thinking that because they're 'burning off their sugar intake' they are not at risk. The reality is that nothing could be further from the truth. At his peak, Steve Redgrave was quite possibly the finest athlete on the planet. He won an unprecedented five gold medals and was the world's best mean, lean rowing machine. No doubt, like so many athletes, he was probably 'sugar burning' most of the time, perhaps filling up on white pasta and rice, and maybe even sugary sweets like chocolate. So, although he never became fat, as he was 'burning the excess calories' with his strenuous exercise programme, he did develop diabetes. Now I must make clear that I don't know if in his case the refined carbs and sugars were the cause of his diabetes as I have no idea what his diet was and clearly when someone has type I diabetes (the type where you have to inject) hereditary factors come into play. However, what I want to make clear is that just because you burn it off on the weight front, you are also burning off the ability of your pancreas to regulate insulin. This is why I cannot understand how Cadbury were ever allowed to do their 'Get Active' promotion. A promotion where they even said the problem is not the food but too little exercise – as long as we can encourage children to 'Get Active' they will burn off the calories. Yes, but they will also be burning out their pancreas and overworking other organs unless someone tells them what's happening. On my travels from one of my 'Ultimate Health Weekends' in Ireland, a very tall, sporty young man told me how he spends a whopping £40 a week on mass-market chocolate. When I explained how much sugar he was having he said, 'That doesn't matter to me, I do loads of exercise.' If only he knew!

So you may be asking, if the government know this, why on earth do they allow up to 40% of this drug food to be poured into mass-market chocolate: a product whose main advertising budget is aimed at children. Well, like so many things in life:

IT'S NOT WHAT YOU KNOW, IT'S *WHO* YOU KNOW

The WHO in question is none other than the World Health Organisation. A body of people selected to look after, not just one nation's health, but that of the world! In 1992, WHO, during their first ever plan of action on world nutrition, spent two long meetings in Copenhagen and Geneva arguing whether sugar should even be mentioned in the plan. Why was this even in question when the evidence against this so-called food was, and is, so clear? Because, just like the tobacco industry, the sugar industry has a lot of financial clout and many influential people in their sugar pockets, so can easily produce an 'independent scientifically proven study' to demonstrate 'no evidence to propose any action against sugar', which is precisely why as this first plan of action for nutrition by WHO doesn't even mention sugar. How on earth can you have a world plan of action for nutrition and not even mention one of (if not *the*) biggest dietary cause of disease in the world? Well, it just might have something to do with the fact that the 'independent' paper on 'diet and chronic disease' which found 'no evidence to propose any action against sugar' was produced by ILSI (International Life Sciences Institute). An institution which, according to Dr Derek Yach at WHO, is supported by many major food companies. At this present time ILSI have 'no policy views on sugar'. To me this is no surprise, but it is a crying shame. Dr Derek Yach explains:

'There is no question that if we saw a marginal reduction in sugar consumption we would be able to start making a dent in the growing epidemic of obesity and type 2 diabetes.'

You need to realize that without the addition of tons of white refined sugar there would be *no* mass-market chocolate and there would be *no* addiction. Before the introduction of white refined sugar, people just didn't have a sugar problem and diabetes was virtually unknown. The chocolate industry, just like the candy, sweet and fast-food industries rely on the stuff, which is why they will continue to try and blind us all with 'scientifically proven papers' showing why chocolate is 'good for your health'. You will probably have noticed that the chocolate industry tries to distance itself from the sugar industry and instead give the impression that chocolate is all about the healthy cocoa bean and 'healthy' cocoa butter. Yet the chocolate industry is the second largest user of white refined sugar in the world (after the 'soft drinks' industry) and sugar, as I am going to keep repeating, often adds anything up to 40% of a bar of chocolate. Every time you have a mass-market chocolate bar you are slowly but surely robbing your 'insulin' bank account. An account, which once depleted, will leave you opening your very own insulin-dependent account at your local hospital – and that really will give you the needle!

There are three main reasons why the chocolate industry adds such a massive quantity of white refined sugar to their 'food'. Sugar:

1 Covers up the foul and bitter taste of cocoa;
2 Gives chocolate shelf life;
3 Makes chocolate addictive.

And, boy oh boy, what an addiction it can be. As mentioned in *Your Health At Risk* by Toni Jeffreys' PhD:

'Refined sugar is partially insidious as it produces addiction as severe as any drug addiction. The only difference between heroin addiction and sugar addiction is that sugar doesn't need injection, is readily consumable because of its availability, and isn't considered a social evil. However the strength of sugar addiction is just as strong as heroin addiction.'

Personally I'm not entirely sure if you should put sugar and heroin in the same sentence, but sugar and nicotine most certainly. It is highly dangerous, highly addictive and it has people with power and money doing their hardest to keep things quiet. Psychologists at Princeton University in New Jersey *would* put heroin and sugar in the same sentence though. Their studies have shown that rats fed a diet containing 25% sugar were thrown into a state of confusion and anxiety when the sugar was removed. The rats had symptoms including chattering teeth and the shakes, very similar to those seen in humans suffering from withdrawal from nicotine or morphine. White refined sugar is not just like a drug – it is a drug and the chocolate industry tastes sweet profits the more they add.

White refined sugar does indeed play a *major* part, in the 'chocolate trap', please make no mistake about that, both in the way it acts physically in the body and the emotional illusions it creates in the mind. However, there is definitely more to the chocolate than sugar. This becomes very clear when you read comments from people like Toni Jeffreys. Despite her absolute hatred for sugar, as is very apparent in her book, the author of *Your Health At Risk* admits:

'… I have virtually lost my taste for sweet things, *except for chocolate*. What I dream of now, is a wholesome chocolate bar made with Stevia (the most naturally sweet plant on earth) instead of sugar …'

This helps to illustrate that chocolate, for many people, is just 'different' to any other sweet, which once again confirms that it is more than just sugar which makes mass-market chocolate the addictive drug food that it is. Remember, there are many, many layers to this chocolate wolf of which just *one* is sugar.

COVER-UP STORY

Back in the 18th century, when the doctors and priests were adding sugar to their chocolate 'medicine' brew there were very few who could stomach it – the chocolate in the 1700s tasted nothing like today's concoction; it was thick, strong, very bitter and loaded with so much fat that many people couldn't digest it properly. The doctors and priests only stayed in business because people were buying and drinking it 'on doctor's orders'. Even then they were struggling and they knew they had to find a way to make it look, smell, feel and taste good. Simply adding sugar to a mass of bitter thick fat wasn't cutting the mustard and something was needed fast.

In 1828, a Dutch chemist named Conrad Van Houten invented a tool which was literally to shape the future of chocolate. This was a hand-operated hydraulic press able to squeeze the heavy cocoa paste, filtering out about two-thirds of the cocoa butter. This process left behind a brittle cake-like residue that could be pulverized into a fine powder, a powder we now know as cocoa powder. Van Houten also treated the powder with alkaline salts, enabling the powder to mix better with water. This process (known as 'Dutching' or 'alkalizing') also helped to lighten the flavour and darken the chocolate.

Although much easier to stomach than the thick bitter chocolate 'medicine' brew, this chocolate was still very grainy and quite bitter. But sales soon took off because it was new, people thought it had special powers and was 'good for you', you could actually hold it in your hand and eat it – and it was one hell of an improvement on the old concoction! Not to the tune of the $2 billion spent every year just on M&Ms you understand, but it went well. Not long after word had got out about what Van Houten had achieved, manufacturers soon stumbled on the idea of melting the cocoa butter and combining it with a blend of ground cocoa beans and, of course, sugar! The mixture this produced was a smooth and workable paste that enabled – yes, you guessed it – *additional* sugar to be added without it becoming gritty. This paste could then be moulded into any shape and before you could say, 'Fry Brothers' – the first ever eating chocolate was born.

However, even with the sugar, although tasting a whole lot better, it still didn't look, smell, taste or feel quite right. Then, in 1875, Daniel Peter of the Swiss Chocolate Company joined forces with chemist Henri Nestlé to produce something that would change the face of chocolate and send chocolate sales rocketing all the way to …

6

The Milky Way

Daniel Peter and Henri Nestlé managed to do something in 1875 which had eluded the efforts of doctors, monks and chemists for generations; they had found a way to mix chocolate, milk and sugar together to produce the ultimate drug food – milk chocolate.

You are probably thinking, how hard could it have been? Surely you just put some cocoa powder in a cup, pour on milk, stick it in a mould, put in the freezer and bingo! Well, not quite. In fact, so complex is the process that the submarine, the electric street car, the camera and machine gun had all been invented before anyone had mastered milk chocolate. The reason why it was so difficult is because chocolate and milk are natural enemies: Milk is 89% water and chocolate is 80% fat (cocoa butter). Fat, of course, is mostly condensed oil and just as oil and water don't mix neither do milk and chocolate.

The innovation of milk chocolate is something to be applauded, at least on a scientific level. But what is not to be applauded is the way in which the chocolate industry, and misinformed doctors, continue to mislead the public about chocolate's 'health properties' because it contains milk. They try to give the strong impression that the addition of cow's milk somehow makes this sugar-laced, egg and flour-bulked 'food' healthy in some way – or, at least, not as bad. However, what most people don't realize is that everything we have been taught about the 'benefits of milk' by doctors, dieticians and the chocolate industry is a complete load of tosh – *especially* when it's poured into a chocolate bar!

'A glass and half of full cream milk in every half pound'

Do you remember this ad? Apologies if you are reading this from another country, but the Cadbury image of two glasses of milk, one half full, being poured into a bar of chocolate followed by the voice-over saying, 'A glass and a half of full cream milk goes into every half pound' is perhaps one of the most famous of all time in the UK. To this day, Cadbury use the image as their trade mark and to this day they are still allowed to use the slogan for their advertising. I don't blame them, as it was the introduction of milk which sent sales through the roof and it is the ingredient that makes chocolate what it is today.

Milton Hershey, creator of the most popular chocolate in the US, knew as far back as 1902 the importance milk would play in building his chocolate empire. He purchased 1,200 acres of undeveloped land in Dauphin County. The land was full of cows and green pastures. It is understood that Milton knew milk, along with sugar would become his most important ingredient, not cocoa. He even knew that his dark chocolate was too bitter for widespread appeal – and it was too expensive. Milk would make the flavour less bitter and, more importantly, would lower the cost. However, Milton didn't cross the waters to see how milk chocolate was being made, instead he chose to do a bit of DIY, which could have proved disastrous. Milk in itself contains lots of butter fat, which can easily turn chocolate rancid. It is believed that when Mr Hershey was developing his milk chocolate he used some milk which was 'on the turn' and this gave it a very different taste – almost rancid, in fact. To this day Hershey chocolate still tastes, I'd say different, others say, 'like it's off!' However, the people of the

US are used to it and the combination of sugar, cocoa, fat, and chemicals covered in what is described by many as 'slightly dodgy milk' still sells by the bucket load. Milton Hershey was bang on the chocolate button when he said milk would be the future of chocolate.

The introduction of Dairy Milk was, according to *The Cadbury Story* by Carl Chinn 'as vital for the growth and success of Cadbury as had been Cocoa Essence'. By 1914 the introduction of 'milk' to chocolate had made Cadbury's Dairy Milk (or CDM as it is known) the firm's major line and by 1917 had pushed the more bitter tasting darker chocolate into virtual obscurity. By the mid-1980s sales of Dairy Milk had reached such a point that Cadbury were handling 17 million gallons of milk every year. Today that figure has grown to an incredible *half a million litres of milk every day* – and that's just in the UK and Ireland!

Now clearly, this book is not entitled MILK BUSTERS and if you continue to consume milk-based products after reading this book (as you probably will) this will not cause you to have an uncontrollable craving for chocolate! However, although milk as a substance is largely non-addictive, it is a large layer of the chocolate wolf and without it mass-market chocolate would have never reached the levels it has. Without milk the texture of chocolate would still be gritty and, even with the sugar, it would still be bitter. In order to strip the chocolate industry bare, we need to remove the complete bullshit we've all been taught about milk in order to help you to chocolate freedom.

EVEN COWS DON'T DRINK MILK!

Cow's milk was *never* designed for human consumption. I realize I may be losing some of you here, but think about it. Cow's milk was designed for a calf – not a human! I know we have been completely Derren Browned since birth to believe otherwise, but if we can all be at home to Mr Common Sense for just a minute it should become crystal clear that not only was cow's milk *not* designed for human consumption, but as an adult mammal we shouldn't be consuming *any* kind of milk. We are the only adult mammals who drink milk after weaning age – even cows don't drink milk. If you think adult cats and dogs drink milk, please keep in mind who controls what they eat – yep, us!

As illustrated with the two advertising gentlemen who created 'their' idea for an ad and slogan with Derren Brown, this scenario also applies to milk. It is not our idea to have milk and never has been. Do you honestly believe you would ever, no matter how thirsty you were, jump over a fence, kneel down and start sucking on a cow's udder? Would anyone in their right mind do this? What would you think if you were driving along and saw a family of four in a field, all under a cow sucking milk from it? Would you think, 'How natural?' Or would you pick up your mobile phone and call the police?

Ever since we were knee high to a grasshopper, everyone and their mother taught us that cow's milk was as natural and normal for humans as eating fruit. In fact, the conditioning by the Milk Marketing Board and the government was so strong that it became compulsory to have it in school. 'Good for the bones', 'Excellent for your teeth' was, and still is, the cry of doctors and teachers alike. No expense has been spared to condition us into believing that we are not just doing ourselves good by having milk, but that we will crumble and wither away if we *don't* have it.

Advert after advert show cows roaming in green fields with voice-overs explaining how milk is a good source of calcium and an excellent protein. No wonder most people are under the misapprehension that the milk from cows is good for humans. What they don't explain is that the protein found in cow's milk is chemically bound to the calcium. In order to digest this properly and utilize the protein and calcium efficiently we need two digestive enzymes – rennin and lactase. Rennin and lactase help to separate the calcium and protein in order for the body to benefit from its goodness. However, and this is a big however, after the age of three we stop producing the enzyme rennin and most people lose the ability to produce lactase – hence so many people being 'lactose intolerant'. What this means is that while we were, of course, designed to drink milk, this was only as babies and only our own species' milk in an *unpasteurized* form. What we are not meant to have is pasteurized (dead) milk which was designed for a species with four stomachs (we have one).

Something the marketing people choose to leave out of their ads for milk is that the protein in milk, casein, is used as a base for one of the strongest wood glues known to mankind. This stuff sticks to the walls of your intestine and stomach. In fact, you may even know this without realizing it. Have you ever heard people saying, 'I'm going for a few pints tonight, but I don't want to get drunk too early so I'm going to "line my stomach" with milk.' And this is exactly what they are doing – lining their stomachs with a mucus-forming liquid designed for a completely different species. What they also fail to tell you is that one of the main uses of calcium in the body is to help neutralize acid. This means that if you have, say, a coffee, the body needs to borrow from its calcium stores to help neutralize the acidic reaction of the caffeine. This gradual depletion leads to a calcium *deficit* which can manifest itself as brittle bone disease, more commonly known as osteoporosis. Doctors and nutritionists will normally advise anyone with this condition to eat more 'calcium-rich foods' – like milk and, funnily enough, chocolate. This is because chocolate contains both milk and cocoa and so, according to them, more calcium. According to Dr John Ashton and Suzy Ashton, the authors of a book entitled, *A Chocolate a Day Keeps the Doctor Away* (no, I'm not kidding) say,

'We think milk and dairy products are excellent sources of
calcium, but did you know that cocoa powder contains more
calcium than whole milk … if you don't drink milk, milk
chocolate can be a particularly important source of calcium in
the diet.'

It appears that Dr John Ashton still believes in the nutritional value
of 'calcium-rich foods' such as cow's milk. Not only has the fact
that we are the only adult mammals who still drink milk after
weaning age seemed to have passed by their common sense, but so
too has the fact that cow's milk has an *acidic* reaction in the body
of an adult human. And what is the main use of calcium in the body
again? Oh yes, it's there to help neutralize any acidic reaction. This
means that cow's milk on its own, especially if you're system is
pretty clogged, far from providing you with a good source of
calcium can even cause you to *lose* calcium from the bones. And
this is without the addition of white refined sugar, theobromine
and caffeine, all of which are well-known to cause an *acid* reaction
and rob calcium from the body's stores. So what Dr Ashton was
doing recommending milk chocolate as 'a good source of calcium'
is a mystery to one and all? He's not the only one either. I read a
quote on a chocolate website from a Dr Weil, *'Chocolate milk is
probably as healthy for kids or more so than plain milk, as
long as it's real chocolate without too much sugar, and
certainly healthier for them than plain milk they won't drink!'*
Firstly, if you look at virtually any commercial cocoa powder to
which you simply 'add to milk' you will see the first ingredient is
once again – SUGAR! So finding 'real chocolate' could prove tricky.
But even if you do, how on earth can adding something with
caffeine and theobromine be 'better than plain milk'? Secondly, the
statement '*… and certainly healthier for them than plain milk
they won't drink*' once again gives the impression that not only is
cow's milk good for us but also that we will perish without it. Dr

Weil says that chocolate milk is probably healthier because, just like Dr Ashton, both milk and chocolate contain calcium. But just because something contains calcium doesn't mean for one second it's good for us. Oysters, for example, contain oodles (exact measurement) of calcium and many rocks are also rich in this mineral, but does this mean we should eat rock if we have brittle bone disease or suspect teeth? And why, considering we consume so much milk, dairy and milk-laced chocolate, have we even got a problem with osteoporosis? Surely if milk, dairy products and milk chocolate are so good for us we would all have the strongest bones in the world. However, that title goes to a mammal who *never* drinks milk and who has never eaten a bar of chocolate containing 'a glass and a half of full cream milk in every half pound' in its life. It is a mammal which also holds the title for the strongest teeth in the world – yes, it's the elephant. Conclusion: the calcium in milk chocolate is about as much use to the human body as a vegan at the annual roast beef convention!

Now clearly I don't think that there will be many of you who, when you pick up a bar of chocolate, think: 'The only reason I'm doing this is to get my recommended daily intake of calcium.' Although, having said that, a well-known author who wrote a book on weight loss (which even had a chapter on chocolate in it), once tried to explain away his eating a Bounty bar by saying, 'The only reason I'm eating this is to get the coconut.' Nut *is* perhaps the word that springs to mind here. I can only assume he also eats Jaffa Cakes to get his daily orange and Vitamin C intake!

However, although you and the rest of the sane world don't consciously eat chocolate because you think it will do you good or supply your nut or calcium intake, subconsciously you do. Never underestimate the power of repetitive advertising and conditioning. The amount of money spent by the chocolate industry trying to convince the world their product is good for you, has an enormous effect. Images of the glass and a half of 'goodness' slowly being poured into every half pound penetrate deep into our subconscious minds. But unlike Cadbury, who have managed to get away with the 'health' impression advertising for many years, on the other side of the pond Mars hasn't been as fortunate.

Mars once made an ad in the US where they had the front to show a glass of milk 'magically' turning into a Milky Way bar. This goes just one step further than the Cadbury ad and, to the Federal Trade Commission, it was one step too far. This resulted in a consent order under which Mars agreed not to misrepresent the nutritional value of its products. As you have probably noticed, that agreement has been about as effective as air conditioning in the North Pole!

THE MILKY BARS ARE ON ME!

'The Milky Bar Kid is strong and tough and only the best is good enough – Nestlé Milky Bars.'

Yes, who could ever forget the infamous Milky Bar Kid? Well, after millions of pounds ploughed into the string of adverts which ran for many years, not many!

Somehow Nestlé got away with this 'look at our product it will make you strong and tough' advertising for years. Once again, like most of the mass-market milk chocolate brigade, they were playing on the false belief that milk is good for you. But even if milk as a product is good for you, that's *not* what you're getting when you have a Milky Bar – or any other milk chocolate – and ASA know this. The Milky Bar Kid became such a success that when they were looking for a new boy to play the role in a new ad campaign 5,000 people turned up – it was the 1970s version of 'Milky Bar Kid Idol'. And idolized is precisely what the makers wanted. If they could make the Milky Bar Kid look like a superhero and persuade

other children to idolize him in much the same way as they would
a pop star, they knew they were on to a winner.

'CHOC IDOL'

This is why, all these years later, even though the Milky Bar Kid has
since long gone from our screens, Nestlé are linking their product
to an idol – Pop Idol to be precise. The UK version of Pop Idol 2
was sponsored by none other than … Nestlé. Every time there was
an ad break we saw a bar of Kit Kat or tube of Smarties with a
microphone in its hand and spotlight on them with the heading
'Choc Idol' in the background. What I couldn't help noticing was
that although Nestlé was sponsoring the programme, Cadbury
decided to do some of their own advertising during the
programme. This presumably was either to upset Nestlé, or to
capitalize on what was an excellent marketing opportunity.
Producing an idol is what it's all about and for years the Milky Bar
Kid did the trick. Adding the strap line 'strong and tough' and
letting the parents subconsciously know that 'only the best is good
enough' guaranteed incredible sales. Both parents and children
were already deluded into thinking milk was good for them so a bit
of adverting, a 'whiter than white' sweet and innocent looking
cowboy kid with a holster full of milky bars was more than enough
to seal a deal.

The success was such that soon after we became the biggest
consumers of white chocolate in Europe. When I say 'white
chocolate', I really mean white man-made chemical addictive
rubbish. I shouldn't really use the word 'chocolate' when describing
'white chocolate' as in reality it doesn't contain any cocoa powder!
The ingredients list on a Milky Bar Chunky kicks off with sugar,
then we have whole milk *powder*, then cocoa butter. But cocoa
butter is not cocoa powder and so in reality a Milky Bar Chunky
shouldn't be called chocolate at all. How they have managed to get

away with describing a combination of white sugar and chemicals as chocolate for so long is yet another mystery to add to the hundreds surrounding the chocolate industry and the Advertising Standards Authority. Robert Humphries was a 10-year-old who got the job as the Milky Bar Kid (1982–7), but even he couldn't keep a straight face when he was shown, in a BBC documentary entitled 'Food Junkies', an old ad clip in which he was saying, 'Milky bar goodness, packed full of milky bar goodness'. He was smirking as if to say, 'Look, I don't believe it either but come on, I was The Milky Bar Kid!'

MILKA COW

There is no question that the Milky Bar Kid made a big impact on the people in the UK, but it was nothing compared to what the Milka Cow did for the Swiss chocolate company Suchard. The Milka Cow and the colour lilac are now so closely associated with it in the mind of the Swiss that a poll of pre-school children in the early 1990s revealed that half of them believed lilac to be a natural colour for cows. Suchard, unlike Cadbury or any other chocolate company in the world, has even been able to patent the particular shade of lilac which it uses. The people behind the advertising used a real live cow and sprayed it the famous Milka Cow lilac for the TV ads. Over a period of 20 years they changed the cow a few times, but the emotional attachment of the nation to the cow was clear. When the best-known of the TV cows 'Schwalbe' (Swallow) retired in 1990 and could no longer produce milk, she was all set for the slaughter house. However, once news of Schwalbe's fate leaked out there was a public outcry. The Milka Cow was saved and Suchard spent 6,000 francs a year keeping her in her old age – which clearly was excellent PR.

THE MILKY BOTTLE KIDS

While we are on the subject of milk, at the time of first writing this book, Nestlé, the makers of Smarties, Kit Kat, After Eights, Crunch, Rolo, coffee and many other products, have been supplying their formula milk free to maternity hospitals in the Third World. Now, before you start thinking this sounds like there's a good side to one of the biggest chocolate and caffeine companies in the world, you need to remember there's no such thing as a free lunch. However, the price of a 'free lunch' isn't usually this costly. Nestlé, according to Baby Milk Action, have been hiring women with no special training, to give out 'free' samples of Nestlé formula to mothers. This usually means that while they are in hospital they are getting free milk, but the minute they are out and all dried up, Nestlé would start to charge them! The reason why most of these mothers don't breastfeed is not because they can't, but because they worry that they cannot produce enough for their babies needs or it is of poor quality. According to Baby Milk Action, in most cases neither of these are true. The biggest problem with encouraging the use of baby milk powder was not simply the sale tactics being used, but the death and disease that was being caused to babies because of the use of baby milk formulas, including Nestlé's. According to James Grant, Executive Officer of UNICEF:

'Every day some 3,000 to 4,000 infants die because they are denied access to adequate breast milk.'

This happens not only because the mothers cannot afford enough to sustain the lives of their babies (due to the massive expense, sometimes 50% of the family's income) but because, in their desperate need to make the milk stretch, they mix it with water. This would be all fine and dandy in the Western world, but the water is often contaminated and consumption can lead to diarrhoea, malnutrition and, often, death. It is estimated that 1.5 million babies die every year from unsafe bottle feeding – this is known as Bottle-Baby Disease.

'I saw mother after mother in the paediatric wards, head in hands, crying beside the cribs where their babies lay, malnourished, dehydrated, sick from Bottle-Baby Disease. It doesn't need to happen. A decade ago we knew the truth about irresponsible marketing of infant formula. Allowing the companies to continue these practices is an inexcusable outrage of humanity, if not outright criminality.'

Janice Mantell, Action for Corporate Accountability (USA)

Breastfeeding is obviously free and much, much safer but companies like Nestlé know that unless they get babies on the bottle, they don't do business. So the real question is:

'Do you love anyone enough not *to buy them Nestlé's Rolos?'*

Despite the World Health Organisation clamping down and despite the Nestlé boycott, at the time of writing this book, according to UNICEF, this practice was still going on.

This clearly is one of the sickest ways in which a 'food' company has sought to generate profits by giving away free samples in order to create a 'hook'. But any manipulation of the truth in order to sell a product which can be addictive and cause harm is pretty sick, even in our world.

THE ICE-CREAM OF THE CROP

In recent years the chocolate big boys have found another way to
make incredible amounts of money from milk-related chocolate.
This time they broke into a previously untapped, seemingly
unthought-of market. One of the problems the industry had for
years was the heat. Sunshine and high temperatures were
Kryptonite to the chocolate world and were enough to turn a once
attractive-looking confectionery into a soggy mess. This changed
first with the invention of air conditioning. Up until then the
chocolate industry had to accept their product couldn't be sold in
many parts of the globe as 30% of the world has high temperatures
all year round and 25% of the rest swelters in summer heat. Air
conditioning meant they could sell all year round. However, once
out of the air-conditioned environment the choccies would soon go
soggy. This changed with the invention of the chocolate which
would, if you recall, 'Melt in Your Mouth and *Not* in Your Hand.'
Hershey, in the late 1980s, even managed to produce a chocolate
bar which could withstand temperatures of up to 140°F. This was
called the Desert Bar and was given to troops in the Gulf War with
the rather clever strap line, 'A chocolate bar that melts in your
mouth not in the sand.' Unfortunately, although it withstood the
heat and was seemingly perfect for the troops who could get
nothing else, it was still warm and gooey. So despite this invention,
when summer hits, most of the mass-market chocolate on the
market today still melts in your hand *as well* as your mouth. A few
years back some forward-thinking newsagents did keep chocolate
bars in the fridge during the summer months, and some still do.
However, these days there's no need as a completely new chocolate
phenomenon has hit the newsagent's freezers up and down the
country – the 'branded' ice-cream chocolate bar.

CREAMING IT IN

In terms of marketing, apart from the initial invention of milk chocolate, this was the cleverest thing the chocolate industry ever did with milk and chocolate. The industry knows the power of emotional attachment and if Mars, for example, brought out an ice-cream bar with the name 'Igloo' or whatever, they know it is going to cost them millions in advertising trying to get people emotionally attached to the new name and product. However, by having the ice-cream bar in more or less exactly the same packaging as a normal Mars Bar, then there is no need. They know people already have the attachment and when they see their favourite bar in the freezer compartment they just think: 'Excellent, a nice cold version of my usual chocolate bar.' In reality it is an ice-cream bar and it does have a different taste to the original bar, but people will still reach for them as they already have an association with the brand. It is no surprise then that almost every well-known and bestselling chocolate bar has now been transformed into a branded ice-cream bar. Take a look in the freezer compartment at your local petrol station and it looks almost the same as the confectionery display.

It seems funny that the chocolate industry spent years and millions of pounds trying to find a way to stop milk chocolate melting in hot temperatures, yet all they had to do was to add more milk, a bit of air and stick it in the freezer (I know there's slightly more to it, but you get the point!). The 'branded' ice-cream bar has proved an unbelievable success and helps to keep the brands' flags flying in the summer months when people would usually shy away from soggy chocolate and reach for ice-cream instead. It also means more money for the industry – not only do they sell more without the need to spend millions in additional advertising, but with the ice-cream versions they can use less expensive chocolate, more cheap sugar and more and more … AIR!

I wonder if that means there's more than a 'glass and a half' in the Dairy Milk branded ice-cream bar? If so, maybe they will claim it's even better for you than normal Dairy Milk!

Combining chocolate and ice-cream is nothing new. Ben and Jerry, Haagen-Dazs and the ice-cream long-timers like Wall's are all mixing 'chocolate chip' in with their sugar-infested milky tubs. And do you know where the company who owns Haagen-Dazs comes from? Sweden? Denmark? Finland? All wrong, it's America! Do you know what the literal translation for Haagen-Dazs is? Well, actually it means nothing at all. It was completely made up to give it a mysterious pretentious Scandinavian sounding name. Did this marketing trickery work? Not many, Benny! Combine this with trendy ice-cream joints, a few scantily clad models pouring ice-cream over their bodies and – WHAM – you've got one of the most successful and recognized ice-cream companies in the world.

PREGNANT PAUSE!

Please understand that when you combine all the milk chocolate in the world and the chocolate-based ice-cream we're talking one hell of a lot of milk. Remember Cadbury alone get through 180 million litres a year just in the UK and Ireland. Dairy cows are deliberately kept pregnant throughout their lives and, because this is such an abnormal practice, many cows develop a very chronic udder infection – mastitis. Lameness also affects many cows due to problems associated with their unnaturally large udders, poor housing and high protein diets (are you thinking of all those on the Fatkins – sorry, Atkins – diet?). It's also worth knowing that a common practice with many farmers to achieve higher milk yield and growth from their cows is regularly to inject their cows with antibiotics. Antibiotic literally means 'against life' and, although there are strict government regulations and regular screening to ensure that antibiotics do not make their way into our milk supply, trace amounts of the drug can seep through. Not all dairy herds go through their lives like this – some live an organic and free-range lifestyle – but I don't think the milk you find in your average milky chocolate bar is from an 'organic' source, do you?

As we've seen, despite the brainwashing to the contrary, cow's milk by itself is not exactly the most healthy food for the human body. The milk fat alone coagulates in the stomach of a human, but once you start combining it with refined sugars, caffeine, theobromine and refined fats, it really does turn into a nightmare 'food'.

Sugar and milk are the two major players in the mass-market chocolate world, and without them chocolate bars would be gritty and bitter and about as appealing as a lap dance by Peter Stringfellow! It is also unlikely that without these ingredients the drug-food scenario would have grown to the extent it has. However, there is a third major player in the chocolate world – fat. Funnily enough, cocoa butter is loaded with really *good* fats and essential oils, but before you get too excited, these 'good fats' are a far cry from what you are actually getting in a run-of-the-mill mass-market chocolate bar. The chocolate industry will try to bang on about cocoa being 'rich in flavinoids' and cocoa butter being loaded with 'omega essential oils' to give the impression you are eating something healthy. In fact, you can rest assured that what you are actually being fed is more …

7
Fat Lies!

Fat – just the word is enough to put the fear of God into most people. It is seen as the root of all evil and is often cited as 'the bad guy' in most foods. The anti-fat propaganda bandwagon has been running for some time now and it appears nothing can stop it in its tracks. In this short chapter I will do my best to at least slow it down.

FAT LOT OF GOOD

One thing I want to get off my chest – WITHOUT FAT WE DIE! Fat is as important to our diet as vitamins, minerals, carbohydrates and protein. Fats are the basis of the body's steroid hormones which control many body functions including the central nervous system, sex and reproduction, the cardio-vascular system and the immune system. Fats are also an important building material in cell membranes, help to cover every nerve in our body, act as a good insulator, and without them the liver couldn't transport numerous vital substances around the blood. Dr Udo Erasmus PhD, author of the excellent *Fats That Heal; Fats That Kill*, and probably the world's foremost expert on the subject of fats and oils believes that 15–20% of our diet should consist of FAT. Yes, despite the unbelievable hogwash we have been taught, FAT IS GOOD ... *but it must, be of the right kind*!

THE GOOD, THE BAD AND THE UGLY

Fats can be put into three categories – the good, the bad and the damned ugly. Society in general sees saturated fats (found in red meat) as falling into the 'bad' category. This is mainly due to the false belief that saturated fat causes high cholesterol, and that high cholesterol, in turn, leads to heart disease. You may now be wondering what I mean by 'false belief', as you may well believe it too. However, despite all the bad press, there is no proof that saturated fat causes heart disease. (Please read much more on this in the new revised and updated version of *Slim 4 Life: Freedom From The Food Trap*). Natural fats (found in foods such as avocados and olives) contain 'good' fats, while refined trans-fatty acids (like those found in mass-market chocolate) fall smack bang into the downright ugly category. Before we get on to the full effect of refined trans-fatty acids, you need to know why some fats aren't just good for you – they are *essential*.

In 1929, scientists Mildred and George Burr discovered the most important fats and oils in our diets – Essential Fatty Acids (EFAs). The reason why they are called 'essential' is because they cannot be manufactured in the body and *must* be eaten regularly in the form of fats and oils. A deficiency in these fats can lead to wounds not healing properly, kidney failure, liver degeneration, breakdown of the immune system, common infections, skin problems, hair loss and a dehydrated system to name just a few. So as you can see, despite the 'Keep Clear of Fat' brigade which has had a loud voice for the last 30 years, fats and oils are essential to our diet. So compelling is the evidence for EFAs that in 1977 the WHO (World Health Organisation), with the agreement of the United Nations, made the following recommendation:

'In light of the present knowledge, it seems prudent to
recommend that future lines of research follow the requirements
for EFAs, that it is desirable that they are not lost by commercial
processing and that the problem must be addressed by law.'

Which is of course a nice way of saying, 'Don't mess with the oil in
our food or you'll feel the strong arm of the law' ... unless, of
course, you happen to be in the mass-market chocolate industry!
And as you have already seen, they tend to be a law unto
themselves. When it comes to 'Good Fat' propaganda, the choc
brigade once again reign supreme.

'The good news is that sensible snacking can play a very
important role in a healthy diet and healthy lifestyle. In fact,
some experts theorize that our bodies were meant to eat this
way. Current research suggests that having numerous smaller
meals over the course of the day helps to keep your blood-sugar
levels on a more even keel. At the same time, "grazing" has also
been *shown to keep fatty acids in the blood stable* and reduce
total cholesterol levels significantly.'

Believe it or not, this statement comes from the promotional
material of one of the largest chocolate companies in the world –
Nestlé. Please note the end of the paragraph, '... "grazing" has
also been shown to keep fatty acids in the blood stable and reduce
total cholesterol levels significantly.' This statement happens to be
true, but what has it got to do with mass-market chocolate? This
is the equivalent of a tobacco company putting a statement on the
side of cigarettes saying, 'Taking deep breaths on a regular basis,
helps to clean dead cells from the lymphatic system which has
been proved to fight cancer and other disease!' The statement
happens to be true, but if it were in the literature of a cigarette
company it would give the *strong* impression that taking huge

deep intakes of breath whilst smoking a cigarette is in some way good for you.

Clearly the tobacco companies would never be allowed to get away with putting such statements on their packets, but the same rules seem not to apply to the chocolate industry. The mass-market chocolate sold by companies such as Nestlé are loaded with white refined sugar *and* 'refined' fats, a combination that *will* cause fatty acids in the blood to become *unstable* and *increase* bad cholesterol. Yet somehow they are allowed to bandy about claims like this wherever they see fit. Mars even had the front to bring out a cocoa drink called 'Positively Healthy'! Not only did it have SUGAR as its second ingredient, but they also managed to have 'More antioxidant power than many fruits and vegetables' plastered on the label. According to Richard Faulks, a senior scientist at the Institute of Food Research,

> 'If you're looking to boost your antioxidant intake, many fruits and vegetables are also rich sources. One apple contains around 150mg of polyphenolic compounds – the same as you'd find in one bottle of this cocoa drink. So from a nutritional standpoint, a better option is to consume at least five fruit and veg a day.'

Mars have now renamed the product 'Cocoa Drink' and repackaged it to advise the consumer to eat fruit and vegetables too. They say, 'Cocoa Shot complements the fruit and veg in your diet, but as we say on the pack, it is not a replacement.' Which begs the question: if this sugar-laced drink isn't a replacement, why on earth should we drink it in the first place?

Let's get something very clear. The mass-market chocolate companies' primary concern is to keep their profits turning over and to avoid being criticized for the unhealthy aspects of their products down the line they continue to bang on about the 'good fats' and 'antioxidant power' in their chocolate. Mars has pumped money into university departments to fund research showing that cocoa beans are rich in chemicals that can make your heart healthy. I'm not saying that there was foul play with these studies, but I believe you do have to question any non-independent study done on anything. What is so outrageous about 'scientific findings' such as this is that when people read big newspaper headlines explaining that an eminent scientist – or 'the University of Blah' – has 'DISCOVERED CHOCOLATE IS GOOD FOR YOUR HEART', they inevitably go out and buy some. But what Mars, Nestlé and the rest of them fail to tell us is that although cocoa beans in their *natural state* are indeed rich in essential fatty acids, vitamins, minerals and 'flavinoids' – all of which are very, very good for you – this is *not* what you are getting when you buy mass-market chocolate.

FAT CHANCE!

What you *are* getting is a *small* amount of dried, fermented, roasted cocoa paste (chocolate) that has been mixed with tons of 'refined' sugars, chemicals, flavourings, milk powders, milk solids and FAT. The mass-market chocolate boys and girls would love you to believe that the fat in chocolate is all about natural cocoa butter, which contains those lovely essential fatty acids that are so jolly good for you. However, not only has the cocoa butter (fat) been heat-treated at temperatures up to 220°C, which can *easily* change the molecular structure of the fat and render it 'bad', but it's by far from the only fat to be found in your average chocolate bar. Remember, it's all about profits and 'pure' cocoa liquor is pricey stuff (and very, very bitter!), so not only do the mass-market chocolate industry pad their wares with loads of sugar and glue-like milk solids, but they also often use hardened vegetable fats instead of cocoa butter. And don't let the word 'vegetable' fool you into believing you are getting something that is good. Once

you heat vegetable oils and fats to high temperatures you turn
something which was once originally classed as 'healthy' into what
can be *extremely* dangerous.

HYDROGENATED VEGETABLE FAT

In order to produce fats and oils which do not turn rancid or 'go
off', manufacturers subject them to enormous heat – anything up
to 1000°F. Hydrogen is bubbled through the oil and forced under
pressure into the boiling fat molecules. When oils and fats have
been heat-treated to this degree, (also known as 'hydrogenated',
'deodorized', 'winterized', 'bleached' or 'refined'), virtually all the
naturally-occurring nutrients are lost, including the essential fatty
acids! You may not see 'hydrogenated fat/oil' on the label of some
mass-market chocolate bars – instead they may put the less
threatening 'trans-fatty acids'. But if the name is less threatening it
doesn't make the fat any less so.

For years the harmful effects of this type of oil have been
common knowledge to the people in the know. The only reason
why food companies change the molecular structure of oil by
treating it with hydrogen at very high temperatures is to improve
shelf life and to make processing and manufacturing easier. The
fact that it can lead to heart attacks and strokes doesn't seem to
bother most of them in the slightest. Hydrogenated oil or 'trans fat'
can easily create a build-up of LDL (low-density lipoprotein)
cholesterol (the bad one), the small LDL molecules squeezing
beneath the blood vessel linings, narrowing the passageways with a
layer of 'plaque'. The process of hydrogenating fats creates
molecules which are forced into shapes that were never designed
to fit in the human body and they have been found to be a *major*
cause of heart disease and cancer. This kind of fat is so harmful
that US government experts have declared '*there is no safe level
of consumption*'. The US are also strongly considering putting a

warning on foods containing hydrogenated vegetable oils (trans-fatty acids).

Think of those small children's learning toys where you have a board from which different shapes have been cut out. Now imagine someone giving you a completely different set of shapes and asking you to try and fit each one in the holes provided. This is precisely what you are asking your body to do when you eat trans-fatty acids. In fact it can be even worse since the wrong shapes often get wedged into the wrong hole which prevents the right shapes from ever getting to where they belong! What this means in practice is that eating hydrogenated fats and oil can prevent beneficial fat molecules from gaining entrance to your system, which makes the chocolate industry's claims for 'essential fatty acids' in cocoa butter even more of a mockery. It also means that the mass-market chocolate companies don't have to worry about you feeling genuinely satisfied for too long. They know that the right kinds of fat are not only excellent for the body but, more importantly, also help to regulate your appetite and leave you feeling satisfied. No doubt they also know that if the body cannot gain access to the essential fats from the 'food' which has just entered the system (food it sensed had the right fats) it will soon be screaming out for more fat once it senses it has been duped.

So it appears the 'essential oils' found in cocoa butter are totally ineffective when they have been heat-treated and combined with hydrogenated fats, refined sugars, milk fats, vegetable fats, malt extract, hydrolyzed milk protein, flavourings and all kinds of other additives. This all adds up to the startling fact that hydrogenated 'refined' fats can cause a fat deficiency in much the same way the wrong kind of sugar causes low blood sugar! An article in *The Times*, 1 May 2003, echoed the views of many nutritionists when it said:

'Chocolate fats will linger undigested in the stomach and cause blood sugar levels to shoot up, resulting in a sudden energy drop later.'

Once again this is not good for you, but excellent news for the mass-market chocolate industry. Scientists at the Rockefeller University in New York found that regular consumption of 'foods' loaded with sugars and deformed fats can reconfigure the body's hormonal system to want yet more fat. This statement is reiterated by Toni Jeffreys – author of *Your Health At Risk* – who writes,

'It is not only that EFAs are essential to health in many ways, it is also that one *never really feels satisfied* unless there is a certain level in the diet.'

Once again this is perfect for the GODS as research has also suggested that fatty meals and snacks may cause people to overproduce galanin, a substance in the brain which stimulates eating! Professor Ann Kelley, a neuroscientist, and Matthew Will, of Wisconsin University found that rats fed on a diet high in sugar and fat underwent changes in brain development. 'The research suggests that a high-fat diet alters brain bio-chemistry with effects similar to those of powerful opiates, such as morphine,' said Mr Will. The scientists found that the rats, 'can just eat and eat and eat – they just don't seem to get full'.

I CAN'T GET NO – SATISFACTION!

Mars paid $2 million for the song rights to the Rolling Stones hit 'Satisfaction' to use for their 'Nothing Satisfies Like A Snickers' campaign. The words of the song's chorus are 'I can't get *no* satisfaction' which, when you start to burst the chocolate bubble, is ironically appropriate to the mass-market chocolate bar. The cigarette company played on the 'satisfaction' illusion for years, claiming in ad after ad that smoking 'satisfies like nothing else'. But what they failed to tell you is that the *only* thing a smoker is satisfying by having a cigarette is the *dissatisfied* feeling they are experiencing because of the previous cigarette they consumed. The tobacco industry could have easily made an ad which expressed, 'Nothing Satisfies Like A Cigarette' – and they would have been right! When a smoker finishes a meal they still feel *un*satisfied as they have a 'false' hunger: an unsatisfied 'false' hunger *caused* by the last cigarette they had. Non-smokers don't have the same 'empty' feeling at the end of a meal. The *only* thing which *appears* to get rid of this feeling is another cigarette, but it is just one huge illusion as it is cigarettes that *cause* the feeling in the first place! Is it possible that the same principle applies to drug foods? Remember, the goal of any drug company is to create a situation where you feel mentally and/or physically dissatisfied. This isn't my imagination either, Allan Gibbons, one of the hundreds of chemists working on Mars research and development explains,

> 'The chocolate in the M&M is what we call "refreshing". It's a less satiating sort of chocolate, so you can eat lots and lots of it.'

Just like the fast food industry, chocolate bar sizes (portions) are getting bigger and bigger, in much the same way that cigarettes got longer and longer. If the 'Nothing Satisfies Like A Snickers' is true then why do they bring out 'The Big One'? After all wasn't the normal size meant to satisfy like nothing else? Mars have a King Size bar and the size of some of the Cadbury's Whole Nut, Dairy Milk and Fruit and Nut bars are almost enough to break your toes.

The very essence of the GODS is to *create* feelings of dissatisfaction in the body *and* mind. If they can fool you into believing that the empty feelings you have are caused *not* by the high-sugar, 'refined' fat foods you are eating, but by life in general and that those feelings can be lessened or even eliminated with a 'hit' from a mass-market chocolate then – BOOM – they've got you! As you should realize by now, it's all about the emotional hook and even if the rational side to ourselves know otherwise, people still 'use' chocolate in an attempt to try and change their emotions. Unless you break the 'emotional bond' between you and chocolate you will either always have it or, even if you muster the willpower not to go near the stuff, you will still spend the rest of your life wanting it. Either way you will not be truly free from it – and getting completely free from the mass-market chocolate industry is what this book is about. Freedom is not only possible but also very easy; however, each layer must be stripped fully. With that in mind, let's burst this section of the chocolate bubble once and for all by shattering the belief that chocolate is king of the …

8

Mood Foods

A young lady sits at a reception desk in the entrance of a large open-planned office building. It's the afternoon, the day is clearly dragging and boredom has set in. She then reaches for a chocolate bar and – WHAM – an entire choir starts singing and clapping their hands, the lady's face lights up, she smiles, and the tune of 'Why Can't All Chocolate Feel This Way' echoes around the building. In a split second the chocolate bar has turned an otherwise monotonous and boring day into one filled with pleasure, song and excitement. Yes, there's nothing like a good bit of reality in advertisements to get your point across – and that really is *nothing* like a good piece of reality!

Chocolate is seen as the master of all mood-altering foods. It appears all the world and its mother are convinced that chocolate has the unique ability to lift you from the land of the doom and gloom and catapult you to a land of bliss. This is, of course, no accident. The mass-market chocolate companies spend many millions of pounds convincing people that whatever emotion they're feeling, good old chocolate can lift the doom from a bad situation and make good times even better. Does it work? Does it hell! But it appears that the 'Pleasure You Can't Measure' and 'Chocolate is More Satisfying than Sex' brainwashing is hitting the desired mark. The situation is made worse by the fact that the chocolate industry keeps grabbing newspaper headlines with their 'independent' and 'scientifically-proven' reports on the link between chocolate and 'pleasure senses' in the brain. Once again, when you take a look at the information provided below the headlines – it's all bullshit!

BLINDING US WITH SCIENCE

'Scientifically proven' and 'Our studies have shown' can be neat ways of producing 'evidence' which can easily delude the public. The chocolate industry love this approach and when it comes to selling the 'health benefits' and 'mood-altering' abilities of heat-treated, sugar-covered, fat-loaded, chemical-laced cocoa beans; 'science' is one of the best ways to blind you.

Here's an extract from an article first produced by the American Dietetic Association in October 1999:

'Scientists at the Neurosciences Institute in San Diego discovered that biologically active ingredients of chocolate also target a substance in the brain known to produce "internal bliss". This substance activates the brains cannabinoid receptors, similar to what happens when you smoke marijuana.'

At first reading this sounds all 'scientific' and statements such as 'internal bliss' give the illusion of 'proof' that chocolate can alter moods for the better. However, and this is a big however, what the chocolate companies (who jump on this sort of quote for a great bit of choccie PR) fail to point out is that you would need to eat 55 lbs of chocolate in one sitting to get any kind of 'buzz' similar to marijuana. In case you missed it, that is:

55 LBS IN WEIGHT OF CHOCOLATE!!!

And even then it's debatable that you would experience anything other than nausea and vomiting. The 'internal bliss' they are speaking of is said to derive from a chemical released in the brain called anandamide (literal meaning – 'internal bliss'). Neuroscientist Daniele Piomelli discovered chocolate contains anandamide in 1996. Ever since then the chocolate industry has been quick to pounce on chocolate's apparent mood-altering effects. But to say that just because chocolate contains anandamide and related chemicals, it has a 'blissful' effect similar to marijuana is bullshit of the highest order. The domestic cat is a *relation* to and made up of very similar genes to the black panther, but I know which one I'd sooner stroke! Just because they are 'related' or 'found in' doesn't mean for one second that they will do the same things or have the same effect. Piomelli states that anandamide is:

> 'An endogenous brain lipoprotein which binds to and activates cannabinoid receptors within the brain. This results in a psychoactive effect of heightened sensitivity and euphoria which is similar to the reported effects of psychoactive cannabinoid drugs such as marijuana.'

This may be true but it has very little if anything to do with mass-market chocolate. A Belgian lawyer once tried to use chocolate as a defence when acting on behalf of a client who was charged with smoking and dealing in marijuana. He suggested to the court, that his client had not in fact been 'high' on dope but high on chocolate. He said his client had eaten a massive amount of chocolate which contained chemicals that mimic the effects of marijuana. It was therefore the chocolate and *not* the marijuana that was the cause of the positive cannabinoid test. As the evidence showed, the man would have had to eat several small bucket loads of chocolate to feel any similar effect (if any). You may have guessed the judge was no 'dope' and the accused was convicted.

The irony is that if chocolate did have a similar effect to marijuana you would carry on eating it until you burst (oh, so perhaps then!) Many years ago I used to smoke quite a lot of dope, and one of the effects I experienced is something called the 'munchies'. And one of the things you crave like mad when you've got the 'munchies' is chocolate. If the theory about chocolate having cannabis-like effects were true then you wouldn't be able to stop eating the stuff. The more chocolate you ate the more stoned you would get, the more stoned you got the more chocolate you would crave. And so on, and on … and on.

There is also another flaw in the comparison of chocolate to dope. On the one hand it is suggested that there is proof that chocolate gives you energy, yet it is also said that chocolate has a similar 'blissful' effect to marijuana. I don't know about you, but I've never seen anyone rushing around after a few joints have you? Tell me chocolate gives you a lift and I might be daft enough to believe you, but then tell me the same product calms you down and I have to question your sanity.

CHOCOLATE IS ORGASMIC

Anandamide is not the only chemical the mass-market chocolate industry and scientists cling to in order to explain chocolate's apparent mood-altering powers. The claim is that chocolate contains some 400 chemicals and they will pick out any one they can to confirm the scientific findings. In their book, *A Chocolate a Day Keeps the Doctor Away*, the authors state,

'One of the reasons we enjoy chocolate so much is because it produces the effect of euphoria after we begin to eat it. A reason for this is that chocolate contains a phytochemical called phenylethylamine (PEA).'

They then go on to say this chemical *belongs to a group* of chemicals known as endorphins (the black panther springs to mind again!) and that eating chocolate can bring about the same feelings as 'falling in love'. The authors even suggest this is why people believe 'chocolate is more satisfying than sex'. But once again this is all part of the chocolate illusion, once again it proves you need a new lover – and once again it is a load of old tosh! It is true that PEA is a wonderful chemical which produces a euphoric and blissful effect, but eating chocolate itself does not produce the same effect. PEA is a chemical which is released *when* we feel good.

A couple of New York psychoanalysts, when treating a group of love-addicted women, found that the women produced large amounts of PEA in the brain. However, when the women's infatuation stopped so did the production of PEA. PEA is produced when you are 'positively anticipating' a pleasurable situation/ experience or when you are actually experiencing it. With that in mind, isn't it possible that the release of PEA in the brain of someone eating chocolate is not, as suggested by the chocolate industry and their scientists, created by the chocolate itself but by the *mental anticipation* of what the person believes they will get from having it? It is worth pointing out that chocolate does indeed have PEA in it, at levels ranging from 0.4–6.6 micrograms per gram, but it is extremely unlikely that the PEA in chocolate or any food can create feelings of bliss or have any mood-altering abilities. PEA is metabolized so quickly that it doesn't have time to take the effect suggested. Sausages, for example, contain substantially greater quantities of PEA than chocolate but when was the last time you heard anyone getting excited about the thought of sitting down to watch *Friends* with a big sausage? (Steady!) If the theory that it was the PEA levels in certain foods that transformed you into a land of euphoria, then sausages should send you to heaven and back. If someone said eating a sausage was 'more satisfying then sex' they would be locked up, yet when people say it about chocolate it seems OK. But why? Because you have never seen one single ad saying, 'With These Bangers You're Really Spoiling Us' or 'Real sausages – Real feelings'! Researchers at the National Institute of Mental Health tested the effects of ingesting PEA by eating pounds of chocolate. They measured the PEA levels in the urine of the guinea pigs and found *no change at all*, no matter how much chocolate they had eaten. Exactly the same holds true for anandamide.

MIND OVER COCOA MATTER

Remember that millions of pounds are spent every year on cleverly thought-out 'emotional' advertising aimed at our subconscious. Whether it's the lady in the bath 'blissfully' eating her Flake or the bunny 'Taking it easy with Cadbury's Caramel' or the Bounty man 'Taking you to Paradise', each advert is designed to sell subconsciously the idea that you can lift an emotion with some 'seductive' and 'sexy' chocolate. If enough people say the same things over and over again, if they say it loud enough and if it's backed up by images on film, billboard and TV then it's easy to get fooled into believing this. It is the 'pleasurable expectation' and *not* the chocolate, which produces PEA in the brain. This is why they have ad lines like 'Have A Break, Have A Kit Kat'. A break of any kind is a pleasurable part of the day, but if a chocolate bar is linked to it then the chocolate gets the credit for the 'good feeling'. This is why the ad with the lady in the bath eating a Flake is so clever. Relaxing in a hot bubble bath is a very pleasurable, calming, unwinding and blissful feeling. All the advertisers needed to do was link those feelings to their product and we are fooled into believing the lady's 'euphoric' state is all because she's having a Flake. They sell the *idea* that you too can experience these feelings simply by having a chocolate. This is why the *reality* of eating chocolate never really matches the *anticipation*.

NAUGHTY BUT ... NOT AS NICE AS I THOUGHT IT WOULD BE!

You get all excited, saying things like, 'Naughty but Nice' or 'You only live once' then settle down to watch 'Sex And The City' (or whatever) take out a chocolate bar (or two) and start to eat. The problem is the idea you've been sold doesn't match up to reality. Most of the time the chocolate bar has been demolished before you can say, 'creme egg'. You don't savour the flavours and are often mentally on the next mouthful while your mouth is already stuffed with chocolate. And how do you usually feel, mentally and physically, after you've stuffed a few handfuls of chocolates in your mouth? Yes, like crap! Where's the PEA then? Where's the anandamide, the dopamine, the euphoria? You may argue that the reason you feel rubbish is because you have been made to feel guilty, but if chocolate is meant to produce the feeling of being in love, then surely guilt wouldn't come into it – you would just feel blooming fantastic. Some people say, 'chocolate is more orgasmic than sex' but if eating a Mars Bar had the same effect as an orgasm there'd be some rather loud noises on the bus or train journey to work and some pretty big smiles.

THERE IS CHEMISTRY BETWEEN YOU AND CHOCOLATE – BUT IT'S NOT WHAT YOU THINK

Of course, it's not all mental; chemistry does indeed play a part, but it's not the PEA or the anandamide. The mass-market chocolate industry lace their wares with loads of sugar, fat and chemicals, all designed to produce a '... less satiating sort of chocolate' (their words not mine). The idea is to produce *additional* empty insecure feelings; feelings which are identical to 'normal' hunger and other normal feelings such as boredom, stress, anxiety and depression. The trick is to make people believe the 'empty feelings' are part of normal daily life and that a mass-market chocolate bar (or boxful!) can lessen the feelings. The trick works because the feelings of anxiety caused by low blood sugar are indeed *initially* lessened when they first have a 'hit', in much the same way a smoker's 'feelings' are lessened when they first light a cigarette. But these feelings don't last and it soon becomes clear to the person who thought a bar of chocolate could lift their mood that it just isn't going to work. Mass-market chocolate is similar to most other drug-like substances:

When you're doing it you wish you weren't – it's only when you're not doing it that you wish you could.

That's because what you want doesn't exist in chocolate; it is all one huge illusion that's been cleverly created by the Derren Brown-style mind manipulation moments and drug-like chemicals masquerading as food. It's the *idea* of chocolate that is so appealing, not the reality. The reality is that mass-market chocolate cannot genuinely help any emotion, but it can *appear* to. Dr Paul Chadwick, clinical psychologist at St Mary's Hospital in London says,

> 'If you get into the habit of eating certain foods to relieve unwanted emotional states, say, feeling sad, low, bored, anxious or anger then whenever you have these feelings, it triggers what *seems like* a food craving. But in fact it is a learned response to a feeling.'

And why have so many of us got a learned response to reach for chocolate in times of low or high emotion? Because ever since we were children, chocolate in particular has been used as an emotional bargaining tool. 'Have your dinner and you can have this "treat"', 'Tidy your room and you can have a chocolate bar.' Even when we injured ourselves as children, out came the magic kiss – along, of course, with the chocolate. One of the most famous chocolates in the US is Hershey's Kisses; a product which cleverly mixed the emotion of the magic kiss along with their chocolate. Chocolate also seems to be used as what I can only describe as an edible babysitter. If the kids are kicking up a fuss, out comes the chocolate nanny. When we were growing up we were given chocolate as a reward, as a comforter, as a way of shutting us up and as a 'happy' treat. This was then all thrown in with Easter eggs, chocolate stockings at Christmas, trips to Cadbury World and thousands of adverts massaging our minds; all combining to give chocolate unprecedented emotional press.

No wonder our brain thinks of chocolate when it looks for something to try and lift our spirits. It has been literally programmed to do it!

WHAT A LOAD OF HOGWARTS

Even famous children's stories have involved chocolate as a mood-enhancing food. *Charlie and the Chocolate Factory* is perhaps the most obvious, but the Harry Potter stories also get a look in. In the third Harry Potter book, *Harry Potter and the Prisoner of Azkaban*, we see chocolate being used as a comforter, literally an aid to help you get back to normal after all your happiness has been sucked away by the evil Dementors. For that's what these Dementors do in the stories, they suck all the joy and happiness from a person leaving them feeling drained and empty. And once again we see chocolate being used as something to bring the happiness back. I know this is only a story and I really don't think JK Rowling has been given any kind of backhander by the chocolate industry, but why couldn't she have used some bright delicious fruit instead? The truth is we all come into contact with our own versions of Dementors every day and the people who make chocolate want you to think that if someone drains away your happiness all can be solved with a bar or box of fat, sugar, cow glue and theobromine-loaded chocolate. They must have jumped for joy as they saw this huge piece of free conditioning in one of the most famous books of all time.

TAKE IT EASY WITH ...

A few years ago I read a national newspaper article in which a psychologist said,

'Eating chocolate has a calming effect and helps deal with stress.'

Her theory is based on her observation that:

'People tend to feel calmer after eating chocolate and high fat meals. It is suspected that it is chocolate's combination of sweet creamy texture and high fat that makes it irresistible.'

First of all, who feels calmer? Those who are suffering the irritable effects of low blood sugar? (Just a thought!) And what does she mean by 'irresistible'? This kind of talk gives the impression that you can never break free from this drug food as it will always be irresistible to you. But, as you will see, once every layer has been stripped and the truth about chocolate is fully exposed, chocolate becomes more than resistible. And what about, 'eating chocolate helps to deal with stress'? Is she serious? What stresses can chocolate possibly help? The mental stress of wanting some, perhaps? The fact is, if you've had an absolute nightmare of a day, stuffing chocolate down your gullet will not all of a sudden turn everything into a bed of Cadbury's Roses. The problem is that if you have had a bad day and eat some chocolate when you are settled indoors to help calm you down, then the chocolate gets linked with the more relaxing situation that you are *already* in. The brain is then deluded into thinking the chocolate helped to relieve stress; whereas all that's happened is you are more relaxed because you are now in a more relaxing *situation*. The same feeling wouldn't occur if you were *still* in a stressful situation. If, for example, you were in the middle of an argument and ate some chocolate, it clearly wouldn't make you say, 'Oh, shall we talk about this amicably.' The apparent calming effect of chocolate *only* seems to happen at 'relaxing times'! Similarly, isn't it funny how the 'pleasurable effect' of chocolate always seems to take place at 'pleasurable times'. This is the main reason why most of the time you, and seemingly the rest of the chocolate-eating world, believe chocolate has genuine mood-altering abilities. You, like I was, have been cleverly deluded into thinking it is the chocolate which creates your emotion rather than the situation. A famous brand of bubble bath has managed this trick and even has the words, 'proven to help you relax' on the label. But somehow I don't think we need a course in pointing out the obvious to realize that if you've had a hard day, getting in a warm bath with or without bubbles will help anyone relax. They have linked their product to *your* feelings. This emotional trickery has been going on for years with all kinds of products, but it works particularly well with anything containing *anxiety-producing* chemicals such as white refined sugar, caffeine and theobromine. This is why I cannot understand how this psychologist can possibly claim that chocolate can help to relieve genuine stress. Has she not read the ingredients on the label?

YOU CANNOT FEED **ANY** EMOTION WITH CHOCOLATE!!!

There is simply no chemical in chocolate which has the ability to help any genuine emotion. The *only* reason why we think it does is because of a conditioned psychological emotional attachment to the stuff and a chemical trick involving blood sugar levels. I know many children who will stop their tantrum or bad mood when they either get a dummy in their mouth, they have their favourite toy near them, or have their security blanket; but this doesn't mean for one second that the dummy, toy or security blanket have genuine mood-altering abilities. The child simply feels *insecure* in certain situations without them. So it's not that they are happy with … simply miserable without! It also doesn't mean that the child will always be happy with a blanket, toy or dummy. If they have a genuine stress, such as being in pain, hungry or needing their nappy changing, you'll soon know about it.

I think back to all of those thousands of chocolates, chocolate drinks, chocolate ice-creams and chocolate biscuits I must have had over the years and I cannot recall thousands of memorable mood-altering moments. My only memory seems to be of always having more than I anticipated and feeling like rubbish. This doesn't mean I never had any good times *while* eating chocolate, because I did. But this doesn't mean it was the chocolate making me happy. The 'pleasurable effect' of eating chocolate only happens at 'pleasurable times'; times like being at the cinema, vegging out with a loved one in front of the TV, sharing a dessert at a restaurant or having your own space for five minutes. In fact, the vast majority of the occasions in which we have chocolate are happy ones. From the 'midnight feasts' which we have as children to 'indulging' in a box of chocolates while 'pampering' ourselves on a night in, chocolate has always been linked with emotionally 'happy' and 'relaxing' times. As most of the chocolate I ate was during 'happy times', it's no wonder that I was happy when eating chocolate and it's no wonder chocolate and 'feeling good' became so heavily linked.

So I can understand anyone who finds themselves in 'the chocolate trap' being fooled into thinking that chocolate genuinely helps the emotions – after all it is a powerful illusion – but when people are paid money to study it and still come up with the theory that chocolate can help to relieve genuine stress, it's worrying! The psychologist in question here not only says it can help your woes, but goes on to say:

> 'Generally society has decided chocolate is bad for you and you must be a bad person if you eat it. But still people eat chocolate because there is some deep-rooted pleasure gained by eating it.'

That's the same as saying, 'Society believes nicotine is bad for you and you are a bad person if you take it. But still people smoke because there is some deep-rooted pleasure gained by doing it.' It is true that smokers *believe* they get a genuine pleasure from cigarettes and that they don't understand that all they are enjoying when they have a cigarette is the ending of an aggravation caused by the last one, but the reason why people smoke is not because they love it but because they are 'hooked'! The reality is smokers are trying to become fulfilled with the very thing which is helping to make them feel empty and unfulfilled – and the same applies to drug foods like chocolate. Mass-market chocolate is loaded with empty calories and so *adds* to any genuine empty emotions you may have. So, not only does mass-market chocolate do nothing to feed a genuine emotion, but, both mentally and physically, it makes them worse!

TIDINGS OF COMFORT ... WITHOUT THE JOY

An extreme case of this is Maureen Young, the lady who was getting through a whopping 200 chocolate bars a week. Her addiction wasn't always that bad. As she herself explains,

'I'd always liked chocolate though I never ate it to extremes. But when I was stuck at home with kids driving me up the wall, I turned to it for comfort.'

But the more she ate the more physically, mentally, emotionally and financially *uncomfortable* she became. The more uncomfortable she became the more she turned to chocolate for comfort! From the outside this appears nuts, trying to comfort yourself with the very thing which is causing you to feel uncomfortable, but when you've got chocolate blinkers on, love can most certainly be blind.

You need to understand that the cause of her massive chocolate intake was *not* due to the depression, as it may appear, but the *belief* that her depression could be helped with chocolate. She never turned to heroin, cocaine or cigarettes because she *already* believed that chocolate was a way to comfort her emotions. Not only had she seen thousands of images of people attempting to comfort themselves with junkie-type 'food' such as chocolate in films and on TV, she had no doubt 'used' chocolate many times before in much the same way. This means she already believed that chocolate helped her emotions *before* things got on top of her. However, she also knew that eating too much would cause weight and health problems and so, like most people, she exercised self-discipline not to eat too much too often. But when things in her life got too much for her and she lost any self-worth she felt no need to exercise restraint any further and so she simply gave in and binged. The more she binged, the groggier she felt; the *harder* it became to cope, the fatter she became, the *more* self-worth she lost … the more she ate, the larger she got. Maureen ballooned from 9 stone (126 lbs) to nearly 16 stone (236 lbs) after having a Kit Kat and a Mars before breakfast and a Twix, Flake, Fudge and Snickers bar before midday (and who says chocolate isn't fattening?).

Doctors will say her chocolate eating started because of the depression, but my point is that she was eating chocolate long before the onset of her depression and the *only* thing preventing her from eating chocolate from morning till night was her self-worth and health. The truth is, the natural tendency with any drug, including drug foods, is to have more and more, and the only things which prevent people from just tucking in until they burst is their health, money and vanity. The minute Maureen didn't care, there was no discipline and she binged!

If chocolate had chemicals which created 'bliss' as claimed by the chocolate industry, Maureen would have been the happiest person in the world. It would be a case of the more chocolate she ate, the more it lifted her depression and so the *less* of a need for comfort – resulting in no need for an emotional crutch. The reality, however, is the complete opposite. Why? BECAUSE YOU CANNOT FEED AN EMOTION WITH DRUG FOOD! (Just want to make that super clear.) If you attempt to feed any emotion with drug food it gets *worse*, not better.

Now Maureen may be an extreme case, but virtually everyone who eats chocolate attempts to use it as either a comforter or as a pleasure enhancer. I say 'attempts' because chocolate as a substance simply cannot lift genuine depression or make a party go with a better swing.

If you are still in doubt about chocolate's abilities on the mood front and you are still convinced that it genuinely helps, let me ask you a few questions. Have you ever been really happy at the same time as eating some chocolate? I should imagine the answer is 'yes'. But have you ever been depressed, feeling low, or upset at the same time as eating chocolate too? Once again I should well imagine the answer is 'yes'. So it can't be the chocolate that makes the difference. Have you ever felt bored at the same time as eating chocolate? Again no doubt 'yes', but if chocolate relieves boredom then surely you could never be bored while eating chocolate.

BUT JASON, YOU CANNOT DISPUTE IT'S SOCIABLE

Here's another beauty people come up with to explain why they eat chocolate – 'It's sociable'. It's funny, but have you noticed the same excuses people use for what people see as 'real' drugs, also seem to apply to people trying to justify their intake of drug foods. Smokers, for example, will say that cigarettes help them to relax; help them to concentrate; help to relieve boredom, they give them pleasure; they act as a comforter and are sociable. But you could easily apply this list to just about any drug, or drug food. The 'reasons' we make for eating chocolate, when held up to any kind of scrutiny, just don't cut it – including the one about being sociable. According to the Oxford English Dictionary 'sociable' means 'ready and willing to talk and act with others'. It doesn't define it as 'an ability to eat chocolates with other people'. It's also very hard to talk with others when your mouth is full, so how eating chocolate or having a dessert can be seen as sociable is again a mystery. The fact is, no drug addict likes to take any drug alone, including a drug food like chocolate. I don't mean alone as in 'by themselves', I mean alone in company. If you have a box of chocolates and hand them around to your guests and all of them turn you down, the chances are you will feel slightly odd about having some yourself. I remember many times at restaurants where, because I wanted to feel better about having some chocolate dessert myself, I would do anything within my power to help sell it to the others around the table. Anyone who was on the verge of being persuaded would get the 'Go on, they do mean profiteroles here. Who'll join me?' treatment. If that didn't work, a few emotional attacks on their personality might just do the trick. 'Oh, what's the matter with you? Stop being so boring and unsociable. Life's too short for dieting. You have to indulge yourself every now and then – it's good for the soul you know.' But I can't ever remember doing this when offering apples around or if someone didn't feel like having some tuna! I mean, when was the last time you said to anyone who didn't want an apple, 'Oh go on you boring unsociable git'? It's not that eating chocolate is sociable – it's just that people feel awkward doing it alone. How on earth can someone who is already out and socializing suddenly become boring and unsociable just because they don't want chocolate or a dessert?

BUT JASON, WHAT ABOUT A NICE CUP OF HOT CHOCOLATE?

What about it? Once again the only reason why you have fond feelings towards this drug-like drink is because of the *situations* you have been in when you drank it. The memories I have of drinking chocolate is either being tucked up in bed by my mother as she stroked my head and kissed me goodnight, or being able to stay up as a treat to have a hot cup at the weekends while watching 'Match of the Day'. And the only times I drank the stuff as an adult was when I would stop in a café in the middle of winter and so naturally it seemed wonderful. The situation again was pleasurable and, as I was thirsty and my sugar levels were low at the same time, the overall feeling was bliss. But all I was doing was ending a series of different aggravations at once. A hot cup of anything in that situation seems like bliss, but it doesn't need to be a cup of hot chocolate.

There have been so many emotional situation links to chocolate for so long that it is now seen by almost everyone as a kind of emotional miracle worker. However, the miracle is how the chocolate industry has deluded so many around the world into believing this rubbish for so long. I'm not knocking those who have fallen for this ingenious chocolate confidence trick, I was more than deluded for ages myself. I look back now and wonder how I couldn't see this, especially when I used to say things like:

'I'm feeling really good today. I'm going to treat myself to some chocolate.'

or on other occasions

'I've had a bastard of a day. Sod it, I'm going to have some chocolate.'

It appears the average chocolate-head is so deluded that whether they are in a good mood or bad mood they will still reach for chocolate. So all this 'I was having a bad day' stuff is meaningless as you will also tuck in when you're having a good day. In fact you will have some when you're stressed or not stressed; bored or not bored; happy or sad, having a good day or bad day, or feeling low or high. The amazing power of chocolate advertising and conditioning manages to convince even the most intelligent that chocolate can give you a boost one minute and help you to relax the next! Most people also believe that chocolate can somehow relieve boredom, enhance social occasions and lift you from your blues. But if chocolate, as a substance, did have the ability to act as a miracle anti-depressant then whenever we are feeling low all we would need to do is eat a load of chocolate and we'd be happy as pie. However, as you will know first hand, this is rubbish!

If chocolate did have the chemical ability to provide anyone with a happy boost or help them 'take it easy', then doctors could save the risk of side effects on 'calming' drugs such as Ritalin and 'happy' drugs like Prozac and instead give out mass-market chocolate to their hyperactive or unhappy patients. And talking of hyperactive behaviour, it is now known beyond question that drug foods, *cause* an imbalance in the body and therefore affect the mind. The fact is mass-market chocolate *does* affect your mood, but not for the better. The high sugar content alone is enough to change your biochemistry which in turn affects behaviour and that's before we get onto the caffeine, theobromine and other chemicals. Many schools have now banned sweets and chocolates from their tuck shops because children are hyperactive, difficult to control and find it difficult to concentrate.

However, the irritation caused by a bit of low blood sugar seems nothing compared to the mother of all moods. Yes, while by now you may now believe that chocolate doesn't help genuine stress, boredom, anxiety or feelings of sadness, you may still be under the illusion that chocolate certainly helps when you're suffering from a bit of ...

9

PMS – Pre-Minstrel Syndrome

Or Pre-M&Ms Syndrome, or Pre-Mars Syndrome, Pre-Marathon Syndrome, you get the picture. I chose Minstrel as it sounds spookily like menstrual. Of all the conditions chocolate is supposed to help, PMS comes straight into the emotional charts at number one. In fact, as many as 32% of women are reported to have cravings for chocolate associated with the menstrual cycle. Now if you're a woman who doesn't get chocolate urges at 'that' time of the month or you're a guy reading this, please don't make the mistake of skipping this small chapter. In order to burst the chocolate bubble completely all of the chocolate layers need to be removed and PMS is one layer which has received a great deal of chocolate press. So can chocolate genuinely help to relieve mood symptoms prior to menstruation or is this yet something else which has been said for so long by so many people that nobody questions its validity?

PRE-MAGNESIUM AND SEROTONIN

As usual there are many theories, but once again the mass-market chocolate industry, along with its 'medical backing', is not slow in coming forward to 'prove' a link between their product and the alleviation of PMS symptoms. This time it's the mineral magnesium

and the 'happy brain chemical' serotonin which have grabbed the
chocolate headlines. The symptoms of PMS have been heavily
linked to a magnesium deficiency; because of this the mass-market
chocolate boys and girls are at pains to point out that their 'food'
can help the problem as it is loaded with magnesium. However,
what they are not so quick to point out is that stimulants such as
caffeine, theobromine and white refined sugar all *contribute*
towards PMS! All of these stimulants create an 'acid'-type reaction
in the system which the body reads as 'stress'. Stress is known to
deplete the body's magnesium stores. The depletion of magnesium
has a knock-on effect which then causes a *depletion* of the
'euphoria' and 'satisfaction' brain neurotransmitter dopamine. If
that wasn't bad enough, a depletion of dopamine then causes an
imbalance of serotonin! Serotonin is a word the mass-market
chocolate industry love. It's right up there with anandamide and is
yet another way of trying to blind us with science in order to
'prove' their point. Serotonin is known as the 'happy brain
chemical' since a lack of it has been linked to depression. The
theory therefore is that anything which helps to stimulate
serotonin levels can help to 'lift' dark moods and catapult you to
the land of bliss. This is where there seems to be a slight
contradiction in the claims of the chocolate industry and their
medics. They say that chocolate has more magnesium than
virtually any other food on the planet, yet at the same time say it
helps to raise serotonin levels; therefore making it the perfect PMS
food. However, it's difficult for it to do both. It is the really dark
(95% cocoa) chocolate which has the high concentration of
magnesium, but that kind of chocolate does not raise serotonin
levels. My research has shown that this is *not* usually the sort of
chocolate women crave when pre-menstrual. They usually look for
mass-market chocolate, which has a high concentration of refined
sugar. It is the high levels of sugars and starches (in chocolate
biscuits, for instance) which can stimulate the production of

serotonin, not anything found in cocoa itself. This is why the women who do crave 'foods' like chocolate also crave chips, crisps, bread, ice-cream and so on, none of which have high concentrations of magnesium. The problem is, and here's where the science falls on its face, if the higher levels of serotonin, which may come about as a result of mass-market chocolate, are *unopposed* by dopamine, then there is a good chance you will experience the primary *symptoms* of PMS. Yes, contrary to the 'science' produced to back up the chocolate PMS theory, it is now known that a diet high in refined fats, refined sugars, caffeine and other stimulants can *cause* the very symptoms of PMS as they cause a *depletion* of dopamine which leads to an imbalance of serotonin. In plain English this means that far from helping PMS there is a very good chance that a regular intake of mass-market chocolate will contribute to the cause!

If the theory about magnesium in chocolate helping PMS were correct then women who eat chocolate on a regular basis should not suffer the symptoms. After all, with all that magnesium going in how on earth could they ever be deficient? The truth is that the reason why many women become pre-menstrual is due to a lack of minerals in general, magnesium being just *one* of them. But to say the body can derive its mineral supplies from a denatured man-made drug food is the same as suggesting Jaffa Cakes are a good way of getting your daily dose of vitamin C through its orange content! Just because something contains a substance does not necessarily mean it is in the best form for the human body to utilize it (as we have seen with cow's milk).

MASKING THE SYMPTOMS WITH THE CAUSE!

The genuine, often very uncomfortable, symptoms of PMS are indeed mainly caused by a mineral deficiency. In fact the body is so ingenious that it intuitively knows that during the cycle it will lose vital vitamins and minerals. This is why *pre* the event, usually 5–7 days, the body will instinctively look to 'top up' its mineral stores. But to suffer the symptoms of PMS the person would *already* have to be vitamin and mineral deficient for this. This lack of minerals is caused mainly by a poor diet and a lack of exercise; it is not caused by a lack of mass-market chocolate. (PMS really doesn't stand for Pre-Minstrel Syndrome!) The illusion of chocolate helping PMS symptoms kicks in when the woman *first* has a dose of mass-market chocolate. *Initially*, because of the 'hit' of sugar which sends blood glucose sky high and stimulates serotonin levels, it appears to have helped the problem. But just like a smoker who believes the first drag of a cigarette helps their cravings/moods as opposed to being part of the cause, all you've done is briefly 'masked' the symptoms.

In the similar way as trying to use chocolate in order to 'solve' an uncomfortable emotional situation, after eating the chocolate it soon becomes apparent that it has been about as effective as a laser lightshow at a convention for the blind in terms of actually helping the problem. Clearly I've never suffered from PMS myself but I've been around plenty of people who have. One thing experience has shown me is that even if you drip-fed neat chocolate into a sufferer's veins they would still get the symptoms of PMS! If chocolate genuinely helped PMS to any significant level then PMS would be non-existent. Not only would you not see any symptoms of PMS but you would see euphoric smiles and noises which resembled an almighty orgasm. After all isn't one bite of chocolate meant to stimulate all those 'happy brain chemicals' which are 'better than sex'? Like most chocolate hype, talk of serotonin, dopamine, anandamide and PEA are simply there to add scientific clout to a very weak chocolate argument. You can come out with all the fancy scientific names you like but the fact is that PMS is not caused by mass-market chocolate deficiency and cannot be cured with some!

THE PMS BAR!

However, this doesn't stop the chocolate industry, and if a scientist in some university in the backstreets of somewhere says that chocolate can help with PMS, then that's good enough for them. So good, in fact, that it has led to them leaping on the PMS bandwagon, not only by grabbing a few headlines about chocolate in general, but also by bringing out a bar with the job in mind. Yes, Mars may bring you 'Pleasure You Can't Measure' but the PMS chocolate bar can eliminate the 'bad mood you can't measure'. I always thought there was no way you could make an unsubstantiated medical health claim on the packet of something full of fat, sugar and chemicals, but again the chocolate industry are different. On the packet of a PMS bar, it reads 'chocolate for women'. Now call me Mr 'You Don't Say' but I would have thought that would have been pretty blooming obvious. But does the PMS chocolate bar actually work? Well, it appears that like any other chocolate bar it does very little, if anything, to help the very real physical symptoms of PMS. In fact, despite all the talk and science about magnesium, serotonin, anandamide and dopamine, there is no proof whatsoever to say that mass-market chocolate can help PMS at all. Dr Paula Franklin from BUPA sums it up when she says,

'For those women who crave chocolate, there is no evidence to suggest that chocolate "cures" or "remedies" PMS … It's not just pre-menstrual women who crave chocolate: many people fancy a bar if they are anxious, depressed, tense or angry. This could be "learned behaviour", carried over from childhood, when chocolate is commonly used as a reward or to pacify.'

And isn't it far more likely, as we've been seeing throughout this book, to be conditioned and learned behaviour rather than a genuine desire for roasted cocoa beans? After all, cocoa beans are mainly grown in the tropics and it is unlikely nature intended all women to swim their socks off once a month to reach the precious beans in order to alleviate their PMS! Do you think it's possible that there may be better consumer options for getting magnesium than mass-market chocolate? In her book, *The Miracle of Magnesium*, Carol Dean, MD, ND states,

> 'Premenstrual chocolate craving is widespread because magnesium is at its lowest around the time of a woman's menses. The answer is *not* to eat more chocolate, however, but to increase magnesium intake by eating more nuts, whole grains, seafood, and green vegetables, and by taking magnesium supplements.'

A change of diet, *away* from foods high in refined sugars and fats, caffeine and other stimulants, and towards vitamin and mineral-rich foods is the *only* thing which has proved significantly helpful for many suffering from the symptoms of PMS.

We need to realize that we are the only creature on the planet who craves roasted cocoa beans that have been covered in sugar, fat and chemicals pre-, post, and during the menstrual cycle. All mammals have a menstrual cycle but what would you think if you heard a goat saying to its partner: 'Just get me some chocolate NOW and no one will get hurt'? Yes, you'd think: 'Stone me, a talking goat'! But seriously, doesn't it strike you as odd that we humans are the only mammals on the planet who have a craving at certain times of the month for what is essentially a man-made product? And isn't it slightly odd that we are also the only ones who have television, radio, billboards and magazines? Do you think that just happens to be a coincidence? Not a chance!

NATURE OR NURTURE?

There is no way on earth that our desire for chocolate comes from a genuine physical craving for the stuff, no more than a smoker's desire for nicotine comes from a natural desire from the body to poison itself. The body does not crave mass-market chocolate, the *mind* and only the mind craves what we believe it will do for us. One of the major symptoms of PMS is mood swings and one of the biggest illusions about mass-market chocolate is that it can help the emotions. With that in mind, it's possible that some women reach for chocolate when pre-menstrual simply because they believe it will help their mood in the same way they would reach for it to help boredom, stress and anxiety. Isn't it also more than possible that some women when suffering from PMS simply get into a 'Sod it' mood and so think, 'What the hell, I deserve a treat' rather than feeling a genuine need to top up on their magnesium? The fact is, contrary to popular belief, the often intense longing for mass-market chocolate has a psychological, rather than a physiological basis – even where PMS is involved. And that mental longing is a direct result of years of conditioning, brainwashing, misleading headlines and thousands of adverts banging on about 'taking you to paradise' or 'giving you a break from the norm'.

At this stage, if you have had your mind open, you will probably have at least started to realize that the mass-market chocolate industry will seemingly do and say anything if it means more sales. You should also have started to see clearly that mass-market chocolate is about as useful as a fish fork for plucking nasal hairs when it comes to helping the emotions. However, you may still believe another humdinger piece of nutritional PR. Yes, in excess they'll tell you anything is bad for you, but the mass-market chocolate industry, along with the sugar, sweet, caffeine, cake and junk-food industries in general, are all quick to shout from the rooftops ...

10

A Little Bit Of What You Fancy Does You Good!

Ever since the dawn of time it seems anyone who's had an interest in selling chocolate has also tried to convince the world that it's not only an emotion-changing product, but that it's genuinely good for you. In fact, long before Mr Fry and others came up with the solid chocolate bar, scientists, priests, and doctors all hailed the humble cocoa bean as 'the cure all'. Alexander von Humboldt, the great German scientist said, 'The cocoa bean is a phenomenon, for nowhere else has nature concentrated such a wealth of valuable nourishment in so small a space.' In 1662, Cardinal Brancaccio of Rome declared it was 'a medicine good for virtually all human ills' and in 1825 Jean Anthelme Brillat-Savarin, the gastronomic historian and philosopher highly recommended it for the sick and weak. But before you get too excited, please remember that back then exactly the same health propaganda applied to cigarettes! The difference now is that although the health press for cigarettes is pretty much good as dead, the mass-market chocolate health press is once again gathering momentum. It appears the 'health benefits of chocolate' propaganda is paying off and we are moving away from the 'chocolate gives you spots and makes you fat' image to a more consumer-friendly 'in moderation it's good for you' one. Please remember this is no accident and the mass-market chocolate industry knows what a good bit of health press can do for sales. They are fully aware that if they can convince the public that it's good for them and not make them fat, they have effectively removed the main reason why people try to control their intake at all.

SMOKING OUT THE TRUTH

A few years ago there were many 'scientific studies' carried out which suggested that people who smoke are much less likely to get Parkinson's disease and Alzheimer's disease. Not only does this piece of information imply that smoking can be good for you – but it's completely false! One of my mentors, Michael J. Fox, smoked heavily for donkey's years and yet he got Parkinson's at a very young age. As for it helping Alzheimer's, how on earth do they prove this one? If a smoker remembers where they bought their last pack does it mean they've managed to escape this horrible disease? This is the main problem with most scientific studies, you have no idea just how many people were surveyed or used in a study and, since there are so many variables, you often end up with absolutely no idea as to the true effect of the product. On the 'Hot Topics' section of the official BBC website it stated,

> 'Researchers at Harvard University have carried out experiments that suggest that if you eat chocolate three times a month you will live almost a year longer than those who forgo such sweet temptation.'

Now how the blazes do they know that? Did they give 1,000 people from various parts of the world three bars of the same chocolate a month for the entire course of their lives? Did they all have exactly the same diet throughout their lives? Did they all smoke or not smoke? Did they all have the same amount of stress? Did they all do the same amount of exercise, get the same amount of air? This sort of 'study' is probably the most unscientific you can get. Their explanation why the people who ate chocolate three times a month lived longer in this study was twofold. The first was the mention of chocolate's supposed 300–400 'good' chemicals and how they supposedly supply the body with a good dose of antioxidants. The other was to say that because people are 'happy' when they eat chocolate they produce anti-disease producing chemicals in the brain. The theory falls flat on both fronts. Firstly, they are referring to what is described as 'good chocolate' (chocolate which has a cocoa content of 70% or above). Many scientists and researchers now claim this sort of chocolate has higher concentrations of antioxidants and so it helps the heart, but it has still been heat-treated and very often contains plenty of simple sugars. In fact, even a book promoting the 'benefits' of chocolate states, 'A quality dark chocolate recipe typically would consist of about 30 percent sugar …' That's 30% of a substance which has been linked to all kinds of diseases – including heart disease! And saying that people are 'happy' when they eat chocolate and therefore produce anti-disease producing chemicals in the body and brain is just a few miles from reality I fear. This would assume that everyone who eats chocolate feels happy, but we have already seen that just isn't the case. As we have seen, it is true that the *anticipation* of eating chocolate often triggers feelings of happiness and excitement in much the same way a smoker's 'anticipation' for a cigarette can generate many happy feelings and excitement. But those feelings are soon shattered either half way through or by the end of the 'fix' when the person realizes that the emotional change they expected to achieve has not materialized. Not only have the emotional changes for the better *not* manifested themselves, but more often than not they now feel worse than they did before the fix. If the theory of people living longer because they are happy when eating or taking something were true, then heroin addicts, smokers and crack-heads would be living longer than anyone else! What the people at Harvard didn't seem to take into account was that not only is mass-market chocolate full of refined sugars and refined fats, (which in no way can help you live longer!) but also it can no sooner lift your emotional state and sustain it than it can improve your ability to breakdance.

To be fair, the same article does go on to say,

'But it's not all good news – the Harvard research also suggested that people who eat too much chocolate have a lower life expectancy. Chocolate's high fat content means that excess indulgence can contribute to obesity, leading to an increased risk of heart disease.'

So the conclusion they came up with is one most people bang on about:

MODERATION IS THE KEY

It appears many researchers, scientists, doctors and others are quick to point out that, 'a lot of mass-market chocolate and you'll be in trouble, but a little of what you fancy does you good'. Cadbury are one chocolate company who will seemingly miss no opportunity to show how a 'little' chocolate can be good for body and soul.

'Pursuit Of Happiness Costs UK £96 Billion.

Money Might Make The World Go Around, But Does It Make Us Happy?'

The above is a heading from a study carried out by Cadbury to identify what really makes British people happy. Now call me Mr Cynical but do you think the end result of this study just might point in a chocolate direction? Ummm, let's see. Report contributor and evolutionary psychologist, Dr Dylan Evans said,

> 'Although our study has shown people are aware money is not the key to happiness, they are adept at spending for short-term pick-ups. Some of the simplest routes to happiness include proven mood enhancers like chocolate [*Arhhh, there it is!*] as well as time off work and close relationships with friends and family.'

A Cadbury spokeswoman commented,

> 'As a company with a heritage of bringing smiles to people's faces we wanted to identify the mood of the nation to see just how happy we are.'

Yes, we believe you, you wanted to see how happy the nation is … *not* do a headline-grabbing survey to subconsciously convince people chocolate is a 'proven mood enhancer'. It then continues:

> 'The report goes to show that it's the simple things in life like family and friends that matter the most and for times when we need a boost then a little of what you fancy can do you the world of good.'

Excellent – not only have they managed to claim their product does you good in this survey, but they have included words like 'friends and family' to keep the 'Caring Cadbury' image very much alive. But if you read through the survey and comments they've actually shot themselves in the foot. Dr Dylan Evans said, '… *they are adept at spending for short-term pick-ups.*' Notice the word 'short-term'. Short-term means just that – usually so short that any illusion of chocolate happiness is destroyed before the end of the chocolate bar! And expressions such as, 'a *little* of what you fancy …' go completely out of the window if you're talking about drug-like substances. How many times have you opened a box of chocolates and thought to yourself, 'Just the one won't hurt', but have ended up having one, two, three or demolishing the box? This is because mass-market chocolate is a drug food and, as I will continue to point out, the makers often deliberately make the chocolate *less satisfying* in order for you to want more and more. Now you may not always *have* more and more, but nine times out of ten you will still *want* more. In reality the only thing that stops you is a bucketful of determination and a pocketful of willpower; but the desire to have more is still there.

ONCE YOU POP YOU JUST CAN'T STOP!

It also seems that when people say, 'everything in moderation' they don't actually mean *everything*? After all I doubt very seriously if they ever include heroin, crack or cocaine into this 'everything in moderation' theory. Yet the fact is, on a *physical* level, the body can actually easily deal with a 'little' cocaine, heroin or nicotine and the chances of dying from such small doses are very unlikely. Exactly the same applies to mass-market chocolate. The body can easily deal with some every now and then, but the point is that the *mind* cannot. The unbelievable amount of conditioning and brainwashing in relation to chocolate leads to a 'once you pop you can't stop' scenario. The fact is that the same thing doesn't apply to natural foods which *genuinely* supply the body with its nutritional requirements. I mean, I've never heard a doctor say, 'Broccoli is very good for you, but only in moderation' or 'Mangos and tuna fish are superb but be careful not to overdo them.' Why? Well it's not because these statements aren't true – too much of anything can be potentially harmful. No, the reason why you don't hear this is because once you've popped – you *can* easily stop! I've never come across anyone with a fruit, veg or tuna 'problem' but I've met thousands of people with a mass-market chocolate problem. Why? Because you can only eat so much fruit, veg and fish before the body's natural mechanisms kick in and tell you you've had enough. But with mass-market chocolate the natural mechanisms seem to go on holiday – after all, let's not forget you can eat it in-between meals *without* ruining your appetite. The fact that the majority of people who take 'just the one' usually end up wanting 10 or 20 seems to escape those who advise we eat chocolate moderately. Once again this fact has passed by Dr John Ashton and Suzy Ashton, who write,

> '… chocolate is meant to be eaten in a certain portion size. It's a food that can be eaten regularly but in quantities that are appropriate. I don't know anybody who would like to eat a whole block of butter in one sitting, but spread on a piece of fresh bread is delightful. It's the same principle with chocolate.'

But it is not the same principle at all. The big difference is that butter isn't usually loaded with white refined sugar and people don't have a desire to want more and more until they feel bloated. Giving the advice, '… *chocolate is meant to be eaten in a certain portion size*' to someone who is hooked on mass-market chocolate is the equivalent of telling a smoker they should just have a couple of puffs instead of the whole cigarette, or a heroin addict not to push the syringe all the way down. The natural tendency of any drug-like substance is to have more and more. Again, the only thing which prevents most people from stuffing themselves with mass-market chocolate is the desire to be slim and/or healthy. This is why headlines suggesting that it will not make people ill or fat are potentially so harmful; they technically remove the person's only possible means of defence. This is also why some makers of chocolate will use any method possible to lure us into believing

their chocolate really is good for you and certainly will not make
you fat.

IT MUST BE GOOD CHOCOLATE – IT'S ORGANIC!

The 'organic' rollercoaster has been running at speed for some
time now and it appears the world and their mother have been
successfully deluded into believing that if it says it's organic then it
must be good for you. At this point I'd like to point out that you
can no doubt get organic tobacco and indeed organic cocaine!
Green & Blacks are perhaps the most famous company in the UK
chocolate world for their 'Organic' chocolate range. What I find
most peculiar is that we have reached a stage where our food is
poisoned so much that we even have an 'organic' range. After all,
by telling us certain chocolate is organic simply illustrates that the
other stuff is even worse than we already suspected! On top of the
sugar, fat, flavourings and milk products they are telling us the
cocoa beans themselves, the very ones which apparently are full of
flavinoids, are a few pesticides short of a chemical factory. Once
the beans have been roasted, fermented and covered in drug-like
sweeteners, fats and chemicals does it really make any difference
on the health front if the bean started its life as 'organic'? Green &
Blacks are very clever at the 'make them believe it's good for them'
organic packaging. All of their packaging is very dark and gives the
impression that *all* of their chocolate is high in cocoa solids. What
is really clever is that they do have an organic 70% cocoa bar, but
when that is put alongside their organic almond, mint, hazelnut or
whatever, it gives the strong illusion that *all* of their range are high
in cocoa solids. The reality is that they are loaded with sugar and
have a much *lower* percentage of cocoa than the 70% bar. This
doesn't mean for one second that they make any claims that 70%
organic cocoa is good for you – just remember it may still be
loaded with as much as 30% 'organic' sugar and have a much

higher concentration of the dog-killing, heart-racing, *addictive* stimulant theobromine. Yes, I did say dog-killing. Where, as with cigarettes, it takes a while for our system to break down, dark chocolate can be instantly lethal for a dog. According to Dr Dawn Ruben's article entitled 'Why Dogs Can't Eat Chocolate', 'one chocolate-chip cookie probably won't cause serious damage to your dog, but if he eats just a bowlful in one sitting he may develop vomiting and diarrhoea.' She goes on to say, 'once toxic levels are reached, the stimulants kick in, and this is when you really have to worry. Symptoms include: restlessness, hyperactivity, muscle twitching and excessive panting … If your pet isn't treated, he could go into a seizure – possibly even die' – well, dog gone!

John Robbins, the author of *Diet For A New America*, believes that theobromine is such a problem that he goes as far as to say, '*Chocolate addiction may really be theobromine addiction*'! I don't really think that's true – as far as I'm concerned it's much more of a refined sugar and fat problem – but having said that there is no question theobromine, along with the caffeine, adds to the whole addictive package. Both caffeine and theobromine are found in *much* higher volumes in dark chocolate. Many chocolate 'experts' will tell you that there's hardly any caffeine in chocolate. But although the percentage of caffeine is low in milk chocolate compared to a cup of coffee, it doesn't mean it has no effect. All it illustrates is just how much caffeine is in a cup of coffee! It also shows just how much is in a bar of dark chocolate.

Remember many hours of debate, many board meetings and many drafts go into making the packaging just right. The glossy wrappers are the chocolate world's shop window and they know just how important it is to make it look inviting – and even good for you.

'FAT-FREE CHOCOLATE'

This is one of the biggest food tricks of the 21st century; put the words 'low fat' or 'fat free' on the label and – BINGO – people will assume it won't make them fat. However, it's worth knowing that 'fat free' or 'low fat' or 'no added fat' (always a good one that) usually means MORE SUGAR. Simple white refined sugar, if you recall, is the very stuff which converts to fat once in the body. To put this fat free nonsense in perspective, you could get a bathtub full of white refined sugar and put a label on it saying '100% fat free'. The fact that it will transform into large hips, buttocks and chubby cheeks once you eat it seems not to matter a jot to the marketing people and advertising standard council.

TASTE THE CHOCOLATE, SKIP SOME FAT!

The most famous of the 'less-fat' brigade has to be the Flyte bar. It was launched in a blaze of TV, radio and magazine publicity – the chocolate bar which had 'all the taste, but only half the fat'. The chocolate bar which said, 'Taste the Chocolate, skip some fat'. Remember, one of the only things which prevents people from stuffing themselves with chocolate is their weight, so when a chocolate says you can have chocolate without '*some of* the fat', people think they can eat the stuff without getting fat themselves. However the first ingredient of Flyte is … go on, have a guess, yep – sugar! Followed by 'glucose syrup' – in other words more sugar. The advertising was all about 'guilt-free' chocolate, but how the chocolate company who led this misleading ad campaign cannot feel guilty is again another mystery.

Not all chocolate bars which have labels saying, 'less fat', 'be good to yourself' or 'fat free' are loaded with more sugar; some are genuinely fat free with no added sugar. However, don't always believe the hype!

'Fat Free Chocolate Is No Longer A Dream.

New Research Has Found A Way To Make Our Bad Habits Healthy'

This headline is from an article taken from the *Daily Express*, 5 June 2001. It's yet another headline from the chocolate industry which tries to delude its customers into thinking what they are about to get is some kind of health product. The article reads, 'Researchers have found a way of altering chocolate so that it does not expand the waistline.' Any prizes for guessing where these researchers are from? Yes, it's the scientists at the Nestlé Research Centre in Switzerland. According to this article they've found that by adding calcium to dark chocolate it helps to prevent the absorption of some of the cocoa butter. The article then says, 'Instead of entering the bloodstream and finally turning into body fat, it passes straight through the gut.'

What's interesting about this is that one minute the industry are telling us that cocoa butter is good and that chocolate has antioxidants and will *not* make us fat, then they come out with a way of preventing cocoa butter from being absorbed so we don't get fat on a product which, according to them, doesn't make us fat anyway! To make even more of a mockery of the mass-market chocolate industry's health claims, the article goes on to say, 'Volunteers who ate the modified chocolate for two weeks had 15% less cholesterol in their blood and absorbed 10% fewer calories than those who ate normal chocolate. They also excreted double the amount of fat.' Yet if you recall Nestlé's promotional material implies that 'grazing' on 'normal' snacks (such as their chocolate) has been shown to help fatty acids in the blood stabilize and *reduce* total cholesterol levels significantly. So which one is true? Who cares? All these scientific studies are designed to create confusion about the health 'benefits' of chocolate. Luckily, there is one group which the chocolate industry has not managed to confuse with their 'proven' studies – The British Heart Foundation. Belinda Linden from the BHF says,

'Advising people to eat chocolate regularly for their heart's sake is a reckless message that people should ignore.'

It's even more reckless when you're talking about a substance that has an addictive nature, so terms like 'grazing' and 'the correct portion size' don't apply. You can throw all the money in the world at study after study and advise people to have a 'little' but there's only one true study on chocolate which cannot be disputed – when the average person reaches for a 'little' chocolate, they will nearly always end up having quite a lot. This is not because they're pigs (the same thing wouldn't happen with sardines!), it's because the product we are dealing with has addictive properties. Trust me, it's not a 'little' of what people fancy which is bringing in $32 billion a year in chocolate revenue – it's a hell of a lot.

HOW HAVE THEY GOT THE GALL?

While many mass-market researchers have the gall to tell us a product full of refined sugars and fats is good for us, some people are losing theirs – of the bladder kind that is. A friend of mine knew I was writing a book on chocolate and said she had some information which may help. Her friend's father had his gall bladder removed and the doctor specifically cited eating too much chocolate as the cause. Apparently this was due to the huge quantity of fat it had had to try and cope with (yes, I was surprised too!). Now the chocolate industry will no doubt argue that he shouldn't have had that much and it's his own fault, but again the product is addictive and the industry conditions people to eat the stuff when not physically hungry, so I don't think they're

completely free on the blame front. Cigarette companies came out
with this for years. 'One cigarettes didn't kill anyone', and, yes,
that's right, *one* cigarette didn't. But it's the knock-on effect to the
hundreds of thousands over the years which are the problem.

In November 2003, it did appear that a major chocolate
company, Cadbury, were about to take some responsibility for the
long-term health problems that can be caused from too much sugar
and fat, when I saw a headline in a national newspaper that read:

'Now Chocolate Is to Carry a Health Warning'

Unfortunately, as is so often the case, the press hadn't quite got it
right. In a statement I received from Sarah Welch from Cadbury's
Consumer Relations Department, she stated:

> 'The information in the media was incorrect in that it stated that
> we were about to place health warnings on bars. Cadbury Trebor
> Bassett gave no statement to confirm the story and at present
> are not planning to print health warnings on any packaging.'

And to be fair, they probably never will. If you ever do see a
warning on bars of chocolate, you can bet your bottom dollar it's
not on there because they wanted to put it on. It could be a
pre-emptive strike to make sure they don't get sued like the
tobacco companies and big fast-food giants like McDonald's. But
you and I know, at this stage, that you've got more chance of being
transformed into a chocolate muffin than of ever seeing a health
warning on mass-market chocolate bars. No, what is much more
likely is that chocolate companies will start putting health *advice*
on their labels rather than health *warnings*. As we have seen, they
don't seem to see a certain irony in starting things like a 'Get
Active' initiative, so don't be surprised if chocolate companies start
slapping 'health advice' on their chocolate bars at some point in the

future. It was suggested in the article I read that Cadbury's were looking into the idea of telling customers that 'chocolate should be part of a mix of foods that includes daily portions of fruit and vegetables'. If they do, the effect could be to link their product with something which is incredibly healthy and could give the strong impression that chocolate is an essential part of a healthy diet. It could no doubt be argued that, on both a physical and emotional level, a little bit of what you fancy does you good. But, as I will continue to repeat, 'a little' means nothing when you are talking about drug-like substances, especially when the companies themselves are guilty of creating an emotional hook – one which starts from when we're all knee high and turns us into giant chocolate bunnies.

Regardless of what the industry says, I think anyone who gets through a large amount of mass-market chocolate every week knows better than any scientific study just how much of a hook it can create. This emotional hook is often powerful enough to enslave people to chocolate, which is a touch ironic given that cocoa beans themselves used to be traded for actual slaves a couple of hundred years ago. Sadly, it seems, some traditions die hard. Slavery is meant to be a thing of the past, but behind the glamorous emotional and glossy packaging is chocolate's most sinister layer yet. As long as they make a profit, it appears the lives of the people who grow and harvest the beans with which the average chocolate bar is made are simply …

11

Not Worth A Bean

'Are there any slaves anymore?' asked Dan, a seventh grader in the US. His father's first reaction was 'No, of course not', but when he read about the conditions in Africa he had to change his mind.

A report from the International Institute of Tropical Agriculture found at least 284,000 children, some as young as nine, are working in incredibly dangerous conditions for up to 100 hours a week for no money whatsoever in cocoa plantations all over the Ivory Coast. Many risk severe injury as they are forced to use machetes and spray harmful pesticides without any protective clothing. Many of these children have been sold into this modern-day slavery by their parents who were tricked into believing their children would have a better a life, earn an honest wage and be in a position to send home much needed money for the family. The reality is very, very different. These child slaves work in sweltering heat and are locked inside a barracks at night. If they as much as drop a bag of cocoa beans when exhausted they are hit until they get up; if they try to run away, they are beaten to within an inch of their lives. Many of these poor children will never see their families again and, most ironically, few have ever tasted or will get to taste the mass-market chocolate which their slavery helps produce. The

IITA report is not the only one to uncover this dark side of the chocolate industry. The true extent of slavery in today's cocoa world was exposed in a documentary by British filmmakers Brian Woods and Kate Blewett. As they set out on their journey to the Ivory Coast, where nearly half of all cocoa is produced, they had little idea of the extent of the problem which would face them. 'We literally walked into plantations and found slave after slave after slave', explained Kate Blewett.

I'D RATHER HAVE A BOWL OF COCO POPS

Slavery and chocolate is nothing new. The cocoa beans themselves were once a strong currency and were often traded for slaves – but haven't we moved on? Aren't we just a tad more civilized? Haven't we grown up, you know … a bit? I must say that when I sat down to write this book, I had no idea that many of the people producing the bean were slaves themselves!

The children working on the cocoa plantations come from countries such as Mali and Togo. Togo is a place I know well as I lived there for a short time as a child. Although my mother and I were meant to be living in a luxurious villa, we ended up living in a mud hut and it was then that I witnessed at first hand the poverty of the region. I therefore understand the desperation of these children's parents and see how easily they could be tricked into 'selling' their children under the terrible misapprehension that they will have a better life. But slavery in the 21st century is very different to what it used to be. Slavery was never good – at all – however the cost of the average slave was, in today's money, about £30,000 and they held some 'value'. Today a child slave for the average cocoa plantation will set you back an average of just £50. These young children aren't even seen as a capital investment and are readily disposed of – once, of course, they've been used and abused.

NOT SO SWEET AND INNOCENT

Once the reports from filmmakers like Blewett and Woods, media coverage such as that in Knight Ridder newspapers in the US, and reports by the BBC in the UK exposed what was going on behind the glamorous external world of chocolate, the sweet and innocent chocolate bubble was in danger of bursting big time. Many people, especially in the US where most of the revelations were exposed, were threatening to boycott 'slave' chocolate completely and, with many children even taking up 'mini-politics' in schools and writing directly to companies such as Mars to demand an explanation, the industry knew they had to act fast! Until then the major players in the chocolate world had always insisted with regard to working conditions on cocoa farms, that 'It's not their problem as they don't own the cocoa farms.' But isn't that almost the same as saying, 'I only sell child porn, we don't own the equipment or location where the films are shot.' But on 1 October 2001, and with the pressure mounting, the chocolate industry announced a four-year plan to eliminate child slavery in cocoa-producing nations, particularly West Africa. The plan was to get the 'worst farms' free of child labour, which included slavery, by 2005. It is almost impossible to know if all forms of child slavery have been eliminated. The practice was so widely used that I would be amazed if it has. The four-year plan looked good on the surface, but as late as 2004 (when I first wrote this book) it hadn't done anything to stop children being starved and beaten to bring you your average box of innocent-looking choccies. I would have thought the law, at least in the US, would have stopped them *immediately* from importing any more cocoa from the Ivory Coast. The 1997 Saunders Amendment to the Trade Act of 1930 is a law which prohibits US imports of products with 'forced or indentured child labour'.

So why mass-market chocolate companies are allowed to import cocoa produced with *known* child slavery, even up until 2005, is a complete mystery. Surely the law is the law, but it appears the G.O.D.S. have almighty power and the saying 'they're a law unto themselves' seems to hold true with this industry. When the news broke of child slavery in the Ivory Coast there was a huge call for all chocolate companies to guarantee that their chocolate was 'Slave-Free'. On 28 June 2001, the US House of Representatives voted 291–115 to look into setting up a labelling system so people buying chocolate could be assured no slave labour went into the making of their chocolate. But the US chocolate industry weren't happy about this prospect and even mounted an intense lobbying effort to fight off legislation that would require 'slave-free' labels for their products. That's right, the chocolate industry didn't want to set systems in place which would guarantee 'slave-free' chocolate. Their reason for doing such a thing? They tried to claim a 'slave-free' label would harm the very people it was meant to help, saying the industry would have to boycott all Ivory Coast cocoa as 'slave-picked beans are mixed together with others that are not', so no producer using Ivory Coast chocolate could state that none of its chocolate was produced by child slavery. But how can you possibly harm someone further who is *already* being beaten, poisoned, enslaved and given just enough food to sustain their working life? The industry tried to give the impression that they were doing these people a massive favour by *not* agreeing to the 'slave-free' label! They also tried to imply that if the public stopped buying chocolate *they* would be causing even more misery for the people of that region, effectively blackmailing their own customers who were thinking of boycotting the industry. This is spin at its best and is akin to encouraging people to start buying cocaine so as not to harm the cocaine farmers of Colombia! This is exactly the same nonsense the tobacco companies came out with for years, 'If you stop smoking many people will lose their jobs' – always good to add a little blackmailing guilt to your addiction, I find!

There is no question that if the chocolate big boys and girls *agreed* to pay the farmers good money for their cocoa and said to the Ivory Coast farmers, 'If we find one sniff of child, or any, slavery on your farm we will NEVER buy from you again' they would soon be able to guarantee that 'slave-free' label.

However, the mass-market chocolate industry appears to have a different approach and seems happy to continue to sell slave-tainted chocolate for a few more years until the problem is 'solved'. Of course, in their continuing bid to look good, they will let you know along the way how much they are helping and how much money they're putting into making sure your chocolate is slave free. Soon after the four-year 'slave-free' agreement was signed the chocolate industry let it be known they have set aside millions of dollars to help African cocoa farmers eliminate slavery. The first 'effective' step is a survey of 3,000 farmers in the Ivory Coast to get an accurate look at the problem. On the surface this sounds as if the industry is doing good and have acted as soon as it found out about the problem. But my *strong* suspicion is they have known for some time about their slavery-tainted chocolate and, just like the tobacco companies, chose to act only when the information became public and threatened sales. Dennis Murphy, who was involved in the Blewett and Woods documentary said with regard to the chocolate industry's survey of 3,000 farmers,

'In the end you may get a big, fat report that gives a snapshot of what's going on, but wouldn't it be more effective just to go to the Ivory Coast and say, "Look we're going to stop buying your beans until you clean up your house here."?'

It appears I'm not the only one with the 'Isn't the answer blatantly simple' approach then! Now call me Mr Obvious, but I think that asking the farmers themselves for an 'accurate report' on whether they are using child slaves is the equivalent to asking suspected paedophiles if they have downloaded any child porn lately! Larry Graham, president of chocolate Manufacturers Association said in response to the bad press, 'The industry has changed permanently and forever.' But, just like their mass-market chocolate, I just don't buy it. With 600,000 cocoa farms in the child-slavery region of the Ivory Coast I just cannot see how a survey or two will do anything to help. *Action* is what's needed and if companies like Green & Blacks can guarantee 'slave-free' chocolate, I'm sure Mars and the rest can easily do the same … if they really wanted to!

UN-FAIR TRADE CHOCOLATE

But even where slave labour isn't used, the world market price for cocoa is often so low that most cocoa farmers are extremely poor and are forced to pay their workers barely enough to survive on. By continuing to drive prices down, the chocolate industry plays a massive role in keeping the farmers poor while we all grow fat on *their* profits. The industry has such incredible buying power that if any farmer refuses to sell their beans at the price set by the chocolate company, they know they will starve and their crop will rot. The farmer is almost meant to feel grateful to the mass-market chocolate industry for allowing them to sell their cocoa to them. The low prices, driven down by the industry itself, leave many farmers so financially desperate that they have almost no choice but to buy in slave labour just to keep going. Exposure of this *unfair* trade-off has led to a growth in 'Fair Trade' chocolate which is a reminder that all other chocolate is incredibly unfair! How unfair exactly? According to a report in the *Daily Mirror* in May 2002:

'Ghanaian cocoa farmers often don't have much to smile about. Certain big-name chocolate companies have been known to cheat them by "fixing" the scales which weigh the bags of beans.'

So not only are the prices driven to such a low as to barely feed
and sustain the farmers, but, if this report is accurate, some
companies 'fix' the scales to give them even less! Farmers are paid
roughly double the amount per pound for Fair Trade cocoa and the
Fair Trade regulators make sure the money goes directly to the
farmers and not middlemen or plantation owners. To them, this is
the difference between poverty and economic dignity.

Once again it is up to the chocolate big guns to set an example
and make Fair Trade chocolate the norm. But, despite growing
pressure, many are refusing to play ball. Global Exchange, along
with many others, is trying to pressure M&Ms/Mars to commit to
buying at least 5% of its cocoa beans from Fair Trade certified
collectives. It is estimated that this would take care of the 85
million lbs of fair-trade cocoa that could *not* be sold at fair-trade
prices in 2000, and probably more, since M&Ms/Mars import
hundreds of thousands of tons of cocoa each year. But even if this
was to happen, it would still leave a whopping 95% of *unfair*
chocolate lining the aisles of petrol garages, newsagents and
supermarkets around the world. M&Ms/Mars, like McDonalds, are
the ones mentioned more than any of the others, but this is only
because they are the market leaders; this doesn't mean that they
are in any way unique. Most of mass-market chocolate companies
are focused on profits, and seemingly if that means a bit of unfair
play then so be it!

DRUG FOOD CAN NEVER BE A FAIR TRADE FOR YOU

Even if we do reach the stage where all the mass-made drug-like
chocolate is labelled 'Fair Trade' (and there's more chance of
getting run over by a number 12 bus with Elvis at the wheel!), it
doesn't mean for one second that it makes the whole business of
mass-market chocolate 'fair'. Emotional advertising and
conditioning aimed at children who have barely learnt to walk, for

a product which is full of refined sugars, fats, chemicals, caffeine and the heart stimulant theobromine, can never be seen as 'fair'. Exchanging your hard-earned cash for a drug food which often makes you feel empty and crap is a very *unfair* trade off. The problem is, just like the word 'organic', we can easily be fooled into thinking the product itself is good if it has labels like 'Fair Trade' on them. It certainly makes the products fairer for the farmers and workers, but it doesn't all of a sudden turn it into a good product. No doubt if the tobacco companies brought out 'Fair Trade Organic' cigarettes there would be many smokers who would be fooled into thinking they are healthier cigarettes. Having said that, if you do ever eat chocolate again after reading this book, please make sure it is at least Fair Trade – at least that way you should, by the time you read this book, also be pretty well guaranteed that it will also be 'slave free'. Mass emotional slavery to the chocolate itself will continue for many, many years to come.

This is by far the biggest irony. The mass-market chocolate industry has slaves on both sides of the equation. Many child slaves are helping to produce the chocolate and many of the people who buy the finished article are slaves to the chocolate itself. Luckily, unlike the real slaves who produce the cocoa, your slavery to chocolate is an emotional one and can be very easy to escape from. Remember, although mass-market chocolate contains many 'addictive' substances, none of them have any genuine hold over you. The real 'hook' is an emotional one and once you see the whole industry for what it really is, it's surprising how easy it is to break free. If the refined sugars, refined fats, the caffeine, the theobromine, the chemicals and the manipulative emotional conditioning aren't enough to convince you, then knowing your chocolate might be tainted with child slavery should seal it. If not, maybe these words will help you in your decision to break free. Towards the end of the documentary on child slavery in the Ivory

Coast, Brian Woods translates a message from a worker to chocoholics everywhere,

> 'If I had something to say to people who are eating chocolate, they would not be good words. They enjoy something I suffer to make. They are eating my flesh.'

Clearly not all chocolate is tarnished with the slavery brush and any chocolate you see with 'organic' or 'Fair Trade' on the label is as good as guaranteed to have been produced without slave labour. However, as I will keep repeating, these brands are still loaded with 'addictive' substances designed to create 'false' physical and emotional hungers which often lead to you, the customer, being enslaved. The whole point of this book is not to get you into buying and eating fair-trade chocolate, but to set you free from the whole business of reaching for chocolate as an emotional crutch.

BREAKING FREE FROM SLAVERY

Fortunately freedom from having to eat chocolate is a piece of cake and as we continue our journey I will show how to make the process not only easy but really enjoyable. Many people think this is impossible and are convinced it takes incredible willpower, discipline and self-control. I remember having a brief conversation with GMTV fitness expert Nicki Waterman on this very subject. When I suggested that stopping eating chocolate could be easy she virtually jumped down my throat saying, 'Don't be stupid, everyone knows it's difficult and don't tell me it doesn't require willpower because it does.' Some people take this one stage further and are 100% convinced that there is absolutely nothing they can do about their slavery, their 'addiction' to chocolate, as they are 'chocoholics'. Not in the usual, 'I'm a bit of a chocoholic because I eat quite a bit of it' joking way, no. I mean these people are totally convinced they are true 'chocoholics' in the 'I'm an alcoholic' sense of the word. People who would go to the nearest 12-step chocoholic programme if it existed in the UK. People who feel that no matter what you tell them about the addictive nature, the conditioning, the bad health side, or the slavery – although they want to stop, they just can't. Chocolate has too much of a hold over them and they have these overwhelming cravings where they MUST have chocolate and they MUST HAVE IT NOW. You may well be one of them. If you are, please be open to the possibility that *anyone* can find it easy to find freedom – even so-called chocoholics. I say 'so-called' because whether you are convinced you are one or not, I need to burst this section of the chocolate bubble by stating quite emphatically …

12

There Is No Such Thing As A Chocoholic

'Hello is that Overeaters Anonymous?' I ask. 'Could you tell me if there's a Chocoholics Anonymous in the UK?' Reply, 'No, but I am one.'

The lady who answered the phone was, and no doubt still is, totally convinced she is a chocoholic. Now when I mention the word 'chocoholic' here, I'm not talking about the *Oxford English Dictionary*'s definition, which is, 'a person who is addicted to or very fond of chocolate'. If that were the true meaning then by definition everyone who eats chocolate is a chocoholic! No, I mean chocoholic as in alcoholic. I mean people who strongly believe that their addiction is completely abnormal and due to some inherent weakness in them, often believing it to be genetic. The woman who answered the phone is absolutely convinced she is a *true* chocoholic. She feels she has to go to Overeaters Anonymous to try to prevent her from overeating and, more importantly for her, eating any chocolate at all. She is following the famous '12 Steps' in order to give her the strength to stay free for 'today' and 'take one day at a time'. She is convinced that her chocolate problem isn't down to the addictive nature of the mass-market chocolate itself, but to her genetic make and inability to control her intake. She is far from alone in her thinking; there are large numbers of people who are convinced that they have some sort of personality or chemical imbalance and strongly believe it is this, rather than the sugar and fat-ridden chocolate and emotional conditioning, which cause *their* particular cravings. However, without sounding too harsh here, there is a slight flaw in the 'Anonymous' theory that a person could have been born with chocolate craving genes – it's bollocks!

YOU CAN'T GET INTO YOUR JEANS BECAUSE THE CRAVINGS ARE IN YOUR GENES!

Think about it rationally; how on earth can anyone be born a 'chocoholic'? Chocolate is a man-made substance so how in heaven's name can we be genetically predisposed to binge on it? If it were true this would mean that if mass-market chocolate hadn't been invented then the 'chocolate gene' person would still have an overwhelming craving for something that didn't exist! I know this may sound mad to some of you but the 'Anonymous' way of thinking makes some pretty strange claims. For example, Alcoholics Anonymous say that you can tell if someone's going to be an alcoholic by the time they are just two-years old (no, I'm not kidding) and they even say there are many people who, although they have never had an alcoholic drink, are alcoholics who have just never had a drink in their life. Now I'm not here to talk about alcohol or AA, but after phoning Overeaters Anonymous in the UK and US, it soon became clear to me the same thinking holds true for 'chocoholics' and so the reference is useful. Call me Mr Get The Hell Out Of Here, but how on earth can anyone be an alcoholic if they've never had an alcoholic drink in their lives and, by the same token, how can anyone be a 'chocoholic' if they've never even tasted chocolate? Now the chances of anyone escaping without tasting chocolate in their life in today's brainwashed world would be pretty slim, but OA do believe that the problem of 'chocoholism' does indeed lie in the genes. They also believe, like AA, that the chocoholic is born with 'chocolate/sugar blood' (how nice!) and will have to accept that they are different from the rest of the population as they will never be able to 'control' their chocolate intake. In fact one of the ladies I spoke with at OA said, *'Chocolate is one of our "alcoholic" foods'*, meaning that it's like a drug … *to them.*

But my strong argument is that chocolate is like a drug to *everyone* because it is the *substance* that is the problem combined with the huge amounts of emotional advertising, and *not* a personality flaw inherent in the 'addict'. After all, mass-market chocolate is the ultimate drug food and the conditioning is second to none. Organizations like OA in the UK and Chocoholics Anonymous in the US argue that, 'One is too many and a thousand are never enough' – just like the AA mantra. And for them it is this which makes the difference between a 'normal' chocolate eater and a 'chocoholic'. But doesn't the 'one is never enough' scenario hold true for a significant number of people who eat chocolate? Chocolate addiction is a chain reaction, one creating an almost immediate need for another. I know many people who are fine and dandy without chocolate for days or even weeks, but the minute a piece passes the lips – BOOM – an almost uncontrollable desire for more rears its ugly head. As Craig – What's Your Flava – David puts it, 'Chocolate's a bit of a problem for me. I can't just have a bit and enjoy it – I've got to have it all. I eat a piece, then I hammer the rest of the bar.'

The *initial* desire to have 'the one' and the desire 'once popped' to have more does *not* come about because you, Craig David, or anyone else, was born with chocolate blood or chocolate genes and is not there because your grandparents used to eat it and so passed the 'habit' on. The cravings and desires for mass-market chocolate are a direct result of emotional advertising combined with the drug-like ingredients of the product itself –

that's it and that's all! All of which can be removed very easily and the process of getting truly free can be mind-blowingly simple for anyone.

I do realize there may well be people who are members of OA, AA, or Chocoholics Anonymous reading this now and the chances are their chocolate blood might be starting to boil. However, it is essential that they, as well as you, see through this layer in order to find true freedom. Don't misunderstand me: I'm *not* saying that people who believe they are chocoholics do not have a problem with chocolate, because clearly they do. I'm also *not* saying for one second they aren't addicted to chocolate, because clearly they are. But I *am* saying that their addiction, or rather emotional hook, is not in any way due to their genetic make-up and they are not 'different' to the majority of people who eat chocolate on a very regular basis. The only difference between someone who is 'hooked' on chocolate and someone who believes they are a true 'chocoholic' is the former believes they lack a bit of good old-fashioned willpower every now and then and the latter has been told by organizations like OA that 'it's in their genes'. And because 'true chocoholics' believe it is in their genes they can NEVER be free.

THE RECOVERY SERVICE!

The main problem I have with AA, OA, NA, CA or any other anonymous programme is that they tell the '-olic' they can never be truly free from their problem and will have to spend the rest of their lives in something called 'recovery'. That's right, according to the Anonymous gang, recovery will last as long as they do. Freedom can *never* be achieved and the best anyone can hope for is a 'satisfactory' way of life, taking each day as it comes. But why do these people have to spend the rest of their lives *in* recovery as opposed to being fully 'recovered'? Well, apparently it's because there is no cure for their disease – yes, DISEASE! The people in the anonymous world believe they have a disease for which there is no known cure. How's that for setting yourself up for a lifetime of doom, gloom and ultimate failure?

Now, of course, most people reading this will not think for one second they have a 'chocolate disease' and would probably be amazed to hear some people might think they have it. I just want to illustrate how silly things can get and help free the minds of those who have been conditioned that they have a 'disease'. The disease we are talking about here would be described by OA or CA as 'chocoholism', but, just like AA, when you ask any anonymous group to explain what the cause of their disease is, they say,

> 'The answer is not clear as to the cause. But once you have the disease there is no cure, maybe once we can establish the cause we can begin finding a cure.'

Excuse the outburst, but … FIND THE CAUSE – WHO ARE THEY KIDDING? You don't need a Masters degree in common sense to figure out that years of emotional conditioning combined with a product which contains a combination of several addictive substances might be the cause. It could be argued that the chemical addiction to a 'food' like chocolate is itself a disease since for some it can just get worse and worse, and it does cause all kinds of ills. That I will go along with and if you want to call the disease chocoholism then fine, but the disease can only be there while you are still taking the drug. The disease, as we are describing it here, ends the minute you stop. Well, not according to OA. They will say you were born with the disease and will die with the disease whether you are still eating/drinking the drug food or not. Don't know why, but I feel the need again:

BULLSHIT!

In AA, people who once had a problem with drink but have since stopped are called 'dry drunks' – with chocolate I can only assume it's 'still hungry for chocolate'! The reason for the 'dry drunk' or 'hungry for chocolate' scenario is because they say you were born with this disease and even if you stop taking it, you are not free but in 'recovery'; a place where you will have to stay forever. The way they know you can never be cured is because if you have just one piece of chocolate it won't be enough. Taking this rationale slightly further, this must mean that everyone on the planet was born with a disease called 'heroinism'. After all, if you were to start taking heroin, then the chances are you would want more and more, but remember if the drug takes hold it's not actually the drug which is the problem here – it's you. The problem clearly lies in the fact that you were born with a disease called heroinism! Now who in their right mind would believe such RUBBISH?

When looked at this for longer than a millisecond, it becomes obvious that the whole 'recovery' theory, supported by the Anonymous gangs around the world, doesn't make any sense at all. Imagine someone falling into quicksand and because they start to sink, they were told the reason for this has nothing to do with the quicksand, but the problem was in the person's genes – they were born a 'quicksand sinker'. Now imagine someone lifting themselves free of the quicksand only to be told they aren't actually free at all, but in 'recovery' from quicksand and that the process will last forever. How flipping bonkers would that be? But yet this is exactly what the 'true' chocoholic is being told and many highly intelligent people do believe what they're being told by organizations such as OA. This isn't to knock OA, or any other Anonymous group for that matter. Heaven knows, they are voluntary organizations who have helped many people around the world. But no matter how admirable their motives, they are instilling a false message into the minds of the people who go there for help. These people think everyone else is having 'fun' with chocolate and they no longer can. They are in 'mental tantrum' *not* 'recovery'! I know it sounds simple but that's all there is to it. They're not suffering from chocoholism at all but of *mental longing* for something they now believe they cannot have.

I'M JASON AND I'M AN APPLE-OLIC

Doesn't it strike you as a bit weird that of all the Anonymous groups in the world, they all happen to be for emotional hook, addictive substances and/or behaviours? I mean, there is an Alcoholics Anonymous, Nicotine Anonymous, Overeaters Anonymous, Narcotics Anonymous and even an Anonymous Anonymous (no, I'm not kidding; this is for people who are emotionally reliant on 12-step fellowships) but you never see an Apple Anonymous or hear of a Dried Apricot Anonymous, do you? Ever heard of people meeting every week to declare to the world, 'My name's _____ and I'm an apricot-olic'? No, I didn't think so! So, why are there only ever addictive *substance* genes? And how come those who claim to have an 'addictive nature' don't have an addictive nature with non-addictive things? I mean, if someone genuinely has an addictive nature they would surely have an addictive nature with everything. Yet these people who hammer home an entire box of chocolates don't seem to have the same problem with spinach. Well, you don't need to be Inspector Morse to work it out do you – it *always* has to be the substance and conditioning and *not* the genetic make-up of the person which is the cause of the problem. Cravings for substances which aren't vital to our survival (like mass-market chocolate) are only ever an emotional hook and you cannot be born with an emotional hook to chocolate – you develop it as you go. Or, more accurately, people can be paid massive amounts of money to develop it for you!

The reality is that there is no difference between what we regard as a 'normal' chocolate eater and what OA see as a true chocoholic. Both are *emotionally hooked* on an illusion of global proportions. Each has been cleverly deluded into thinking their lives are in some way *incomplete* without chocolate and therefore *both* are fearful of letting go of their emotional attachment to chocolate. But the 'chocoholic', who has sought help with a group such as OA, really does believe *they* are the problem and not the mass-market chocolate. Mind you, where chocoholics think it's them because of something they inherited, the 'normal' chocolate eater thinks it's them because of their personality and lack of willpower. Both have missed the point – it's the combination of massive emotional advertising and the drug-like chocolate itself which causes the problem – not them. Glad that's finally clear!

IF YOU HAVE TO EXERCISE CONTROL, YOU'RE NOT IN CONTROL

The biggest distinction that OA come up with to try to distinguish the true chocoholic from the regular person who eats chocolate on a regular basis is that they say a chocoholic cannot control their intake, whereas a 'normal' chocolate eater can. In other words 'normal' chocolate eaters are free to eat chocolate whereas chocoholics can never be free to eat it. On the surface this sounds a fair enough distinction but what they fail to understand is that the majority of people who consume chocolate on a regular basis have to exercise degrees of control. Remember, if you have to exercise control you cannot truly be in control and you are not 'free' to eat chocolate. In fact, using the word 'free' and a drug food such as mass-market chocolate in the same sentence is a contradiction in terms. To think about it rationally, if people were genuinely free to eat the stuff, this book wouldn't even exist! The whole point of the emotional conditioning and drug-like substances in chocolate is to *remove* your true freedom of choice. The idea is to manipulate your emotions and sugar levels in order to create the *illusion* that you are free to eat chocolate and that you are in control. This is by far the cleverest part of the chocolate trap – most people don't think for one second they are what OA describes as true chocoholics and they really believe it is their choice to eat chocolate every time they have it. They may feel they lack a little discipline here and there, but it's always their choice. But as illustrated with the Derren Brown and the two advertising gurus, it is an *illusion* of choice. I know I've repeated this particular point over and over again but this is deliberate; you need to realize that most people are in exactly the same chocolate boat. Most people, although they don't give in to their desires all the time, *do* have to exercise control to some degree over their intake of chocolate and that is why they seek help with books like this.

Maureen Young (the 200 chocolate-bars-a-week woman) clearly *appears* different to most, and from the outside people would call her a *true* chocoholic. But she's not a chocoholic, she is simply *more* emotionally attached than most due to her emotional state, and because her self-worth has gone; she doesn't even attempt to control it any more. The problem is that she is probably being told by many people she is a true chocoholic and so she may end up believing that for *her* there is no help other than a trip to Chocoholics Anonymous. The irony is that it is often the people who eat chocolate themselves who are the first to point out that someone else has a problem. One way to try to justify your intake of any drug-like substance is continually to attempt to prove you're in control. The easiest way to do this is to point out all those who clearly have lost the will to control. However, if you're in quicksand but only up to your ankles and you see someone 'up to their neck in it', it doesn't mean you're not right in it – you're just sinking at a slower rate. The majority of chocolate addicts are sinking at the same speed and so they don't even realize they are in it. It's only when something happens – like when Maureen went into a severe state of depression – which the rate of descent increases. When it does, that person receives the 'olic' label and are told they have a disease. Maureen Young reached the stage where she was hiding wrappers in her baby's nappies so her husband wouldn't find them. Again, this sounds like she has a severe and abnormal problem: hiding chocolate wrappers is like an alcoholic hiding bottles. But Maureen is hardly alone here, is she? I used to hide chocolate wrappers all the time. OK, not in my baby's nappy, but if you had taken a look down the back of my car seat on any given day you would have found an array of empty Caramel and Snickers wrappers. I wasn't really hiding them from other people, it was more from myself. Again if hiding wrappers, or scoffing a few chocolates when people are out of sight, is proof of chocoholism, then once again everyone who eats chocolate must have the disease!

SECRET EATING – FAT CHANCE!

Unlike smoking, it's hard to keep eating chocolate secretly. You may think you've pulled this off a few times, but it's not that easy. Sure you may be able to hide the wrappers and even brush your teeth to get rid of the chocolate taste, but unlike nicotine, the effects are quite visible. Maureen may have successfully hidden all the wrappers – and even managed to hide her bank statements showing the huge amount of money she was spending on the dark stuff – but after putting on 7 stone in weight, her secret was out!

The actress Hélène Mahieu is someone else who strongly believes she is 'different' to everyone else when it comes to chocolate, and again on the surface it does appear so. She used to get up and have two large spoonfuls of chocolate in milk every morning, followed mid-morning by a chocolate bar, two large pieces of dark chocolate early afternoon; six–seven slices of bread with chocolate spread a bit later and plenty more choccie bits after that. She would often get what people in France refer to as a 'liver crisis'. This, she says, is where she would go off all food, including chocolate, and then throw up for a couple of days (lovely!). But as soon as it was over, she was back on the chocolate. Her chocolate problem was so bad and her liver crises happening so often that she was told by her doctor that the chocolate had to go for the sake of her health (which seems odd considering the chocolate companies tell us how 'healthy' their 'food' is). Hélène said,

> 'This was devastating news and it took me all of my will not to have chocolate. I was barking at people, it was horrible. You get nervous because you don't have it and you think about it all the time – that's an addiction I think.'

And yes it is, but it's not unique to Hélène and this still doesn't mean the problem has anything to do with her genes or yours and it certainly doesn't mean you're a chocoholic. It is true that the majority of people don't have chocolate from morning till night, but just because most people exercise control over the amount of chocolate they eat (most of the time) that doesn't mean they don't have a problem with it. What Hélène, Maureen and other self-confessed chocoholics fail to see is that even if the 'normal average' chocolate eater was told by their doctor 'no more chocolate ever *again*', for whatever reason, *most* would have to use all their will not to have it and most would think about it all the time and bark at people (or at least want to!). This is because the chocolate companies have managed to get them hooked almost without anyone talking about it or realizing it.

During the BBC documentary, 'Food Junkies', Hélène said, 'If someone puts chocolate under my nose I will eat it' to which the interviewer said, 'as will most of us!' And that's about the strength of it. *Most* people are, to various degrees, hooked on chocolate and *most* people would not just struggle to break completely free, but wouldn't even contemplate it.

This is why the majority of chocolate addicts, in order to prove to themselves that they don't have a problem, opt for a solution which, ironically, proves they do. When your chocolate levels are creeping up just a little too high or your waistline is expanding too rapidly it's time to take a deep breath, take a leap of faith and jump on …

13

The Chocolate Wagon Wheel

Yes, when things get too much on the chocolate front, it's time to go on the wagon – the 'chocolate wagon' to be precise. The reason I chose 'chocolate wagon wheel' as the chapter title is not simply because Wagon Wheels are a type of chocolate, but more importantly because by going on the chocolate wagon, you end up going round in circles.

The thought of getting rid of chocolate forever is usually so scary that it's something the average chocolate eater/addict won't even contemplate. So instead they spend a lot of their life on what amounts to the chocolate wagon or making attempts to reduce their intake by cutting down. I did this for years. In an attempt to prove chocolate wasn't a problem for me, I would exercise control over it by going on the chocolate wagon for a week or one month. This, I believed, would not only prove that I could control it, but it would help lessen my desire for it and so prove that I didn't have a problem with chocolate at all. But, as you've probably discovered yourself, the need to go on the chocolate wagon at all only proves that you already have a problem, and when you do, the desire for chocolate, far from getting less, is increased tenfold! Even a chain-chocolate eater (you know, like a chain-smoker) can go for periods of not eating chocolate where it doesn't bother them at all, but the minute anyone says, 'No more', chocolate all of a sudden becomes more precious than gold itself and then the mother of all mental battle commences. The problem is, even if you do somehow possess the discipline to 'deny' yourself and manage to 'hang on in there' for the entire chocolate wagon journey, in reality you've done nothing to get rid of your mental desire for chocolate. In fact, far from helping yourself, you've *increased* the problem. Remember, the 'hook' for chocolate is virtually all psychological, so the 'hook' actually becomes *greater* when you're on the chocolate wagon. If you feel you are being denied then the longer you are on the chocolate wagon the *more* and *more* precious chocolate becomes and so the desire and emotional attachment for the substance goes *up*. And when the chocolate wagon period is over, how do you celebrate the fact you've done so well and been so good? Yes, you eat loads and loads of … CHOCOLATE!

FALLING OFF THE WAGON

The chocolate wagon also creates a further problem; it *falsely* gives the impression to your subconscious and conscious mind that life without chocolate sucks, which in turn gives the *false* impression that life with chocolate is simply wonderful. But it's not that life *with* chocolate is so great, it's just that you feel so blooming miserable when you are 'denying' yourself while on the wagon. At the end of the allotted wagon journey, the first bit of chocolate seems like the Seven Wonders of the World rolled into one. This is because you've created such a mental aggravation for so long, that when it finally comes to an end it is a huge mental release. Much of the perceived pleasure when coming off the chocolate wagon is created *before* you eat any chocolate; just knowing you now *can* have some is enough to release your mind from the chocolate tug-of-war. This release is, of course, pleasurable, but it's the ending of an aggravation, akin to stopping hitting yourself over the head with a mallet!

The biggest irony, though, remains the illusion that by managing to go without chocolate or 'cut down' on it for any length of time is in some way proof of control. But it's the having to control at all which shows you're not in control. Confused? Let me explain.

A friend of mine once 'gave up' chocolate for a month. One of the reasons she went on the chocolate wagon was to prove she didn't have a problem with chocolate and could, as she told herself, simply take it or leave it. But during that month she was making more than a meal of how 'good' she was being and how 'well' she was doing. I remember her 'holier than thou' attitude and how amazing, not just she, but all the people around her thought she was being by managing to go without chocolate for a month. However, by thinking she was 'being good', 'doing well' and 'being amazing' is proof alone that she *does* have a problem with chocolate. Think about it – if she really could take it or leave it then what's the big deal and why the song and dance? Why does she, or anyone for that matter, think they're superhuman for managing to stay 'choc free' for a week or a month if they *don't* have a problem with it? If I said to you, 'I've been without sardines for a month' would you be impressed? NO! But the mere fact that virtually anyone can relate and empathize with people who either try to give up chocolate altogether or go on the chocolate wagon for any length of time proves that the *majority* of people do indeed have a huge emotional attachment to chocolate and *all* find it difficult to control their intake or get free.

Once again this doesn't happen with foods like sardines, and this should show us that chocolate isn't a food but a drug cleverly wrapped up as food. By jumping on the chocolate wagon, far from showing yourself and others that you are *in* control and don't have a problem, you are in reality doing the complete opposite.

WEEKENDS ONLY PLEASE

Because mass-market chocolate can be so highly addictive, people will often set themselves chocolate rules in an attempt to make sure they don't overdo it. For example, many have a strict rule of 'no chocolate during the week', for others it's 'only one bar a day', but as before the restrictions people put on themselves prove that there is a problem. Imagine offering someone an apple and getting the reply, 'No thanks, not during the week – I only allow myself apples at weekends', what would you think? Yes – they've got an apple problem! You never hear of people needing to restrict their intake of carrots, spinach, peaches or pineapple. This is because these foods are *genuine* and when you eat some you don't have this almost insatiable need to keep going until you feel bloated or sick.

This is why Overeaters Anonymous have it wrong when it comes to their definition of what sets chocoholics apart from 'normal' chocolate eaters/addicts. They are under the misapprehension that the majority of people *don't* exercise control over their intake of chocolate and don't have chocolate binges. But the reality is that the *majority* of people who eat chocolate are always trying to control their intake to varying degrees and many people *do* have chocolate binges. This does not mean for one second that they need to attend weekly meetings in order to declare, 'I'm _____ and I'm a chocoholic.' In fact, they have exactly the same problem with this drug-like substance as *most* other people. The main difference is most people either joke about it – 'I'm a chocoholic, ha ha' – to give the impression that it's really not a problem, or they don't talk about it at all thinking they are different to everyone else. (And others are too busy hiding their discarded wrappers behind their car seat to talk about it – yes, I know!)

The actress Hélène Mahieu says she is now past the severe chocoholic stage in her life and now has a healthy relationship with chocolate because in her words,

'I can control it better, but I have to control it, I do.'

She says she still has to avoid the chocolate aisle in supermarkets, tries never to buy it and if she looks at chocolate she 'has to eat it'. Now call me Mr Bleeding Obvious but how on earth is that a healthy relationship with chocolate? Sorry, using the expression 'healthy relationship' and 'chocolate' in the same sentence is a contradiction in terms. With chocolate the relationship can never be healthy, not simply because the product itself is full of addictive refined fats and sugars, but because in this relationship chocolate, and the industry at the back of it, are always ultimately wearing the trousers.

You may think by going on the occasional chocolate wagon or managing to 'cut down' at times that you are in control. But as I'm sure you must know by now, *they* control your thoughts, your body's chemical feelings and, if things get really bad, your bank balance when it comes to chocolate. The illusion of control is one of the beauties of the chocolate trap. Funny enough, the 'hook' is often so subtle that the vast majority of people who eat chocolate aren't even aware that they're 'hooked' at all until they make an attempt to stop or cut down. However, for those who are aware that they are in the trap, it often doesn't do anything to help the actual process of escaping. So how do we finally kick chocolate from our lives easily?

BREAKING UP IS HARD TO DO ... OR IS IT?

We have already seen that the 'recovery' method, in terms of helping people to freedom, is about as effective as a chocolate fireguard! It also makes a huge meal out of something which can be mind-blowingly easy. On top of this it turns someone who thought they had a bit of a chocolate problem into someone who believes they were born with an incurable disease – nice! We have also seen that jumping on the chocolate wagon *increases* the desire for chocolate, proves the person is *not* in control and leaves people counting the days waiting for their 'sacrifice' to come to an end. All of this only adds up to the biggest illusion of them all when it comes to this drug food – it's difficult to break free.

Now clearly most people don't think their addiction is bad enough to go down the OA 'recovery' 12-step route, but they still believe giving up chocolate is very, very difficult and will *always* take incredible discipline and willpower to achieve. Luckily, nothing could be further from the truth – when you finally see beneath every layer of the chocolate wolf and are armed with the mental route map to chocolate freedom, breaking up from chocolate is *very* easy to do. The only reason why people like Nicki Waterman (who jumped down my throat at the mere suggestion that it could be easy) and all those who have attended OA or leapt on the chocolate wagon are convinced that it is hard is because they believe that it all comes down to willpower. But, like so many aspects of the chocolate trap, the complete opposite is true. The saying is 'where there's a will there's a way', but with drugs things work slightly differently and in the case of chocolate …

14

Where There's A Will
– There's *No* Way

Willpower – you either have it or you don't. Personally, I have about as much as a nymph in a brothel! Fortunately, it doesn't matter if you possess bundles of the stuff or whether you're well under-furnished in the willpower department; the fact is that it requires no willpower at all to break free. Now, before you start choking on your Curly Wurly, thinking I'm off my chocolate rocker for making such a suggestion, hear me out. I'm not saying that the willpower way isn't the usual approach people adopt when trying to kick chocolate, but if you expect your *will* to *power* you to freedom you need to think again. Not only is using your will to fight your desire for chocolate an extremely hard way of going about it, but the chances of succeeding are about the same as flying to the moon on a Flyte bar! In fact, the actual percentage of people achieving their goal using this method is the same as with diets in general:

95% FAILURE!

So why does using willpower have such little success when there are so many strong-willed people around? You may even think of yourself as fairly strong-willed with other things in your life but for some reason when it comes to chocolate you find your willpower melts like a Magnum in Dubai. Well, the answer, somewhat strangely, is that it is the strong-willed people who usually have such difficulty trying to stop when using willpower. Confused? Let me explain.

Imagine two chocolate-loving people, one strong-willed and the other weak-willed, each with a chocolate bar in their hand ready to eat it. If you were to take the chocolate off them and tell them they can't have it, who do you think would kick up more of a fuss? Yes – the *strong*-willed one. Strong-willed people hate being told what to do by anyone, including themselves, and they hate feeling deprived. This is why a *strong*-willed person will actually give in much quicker. However, imagine the scenario but this time neither of them had any desire for the chocolate at all. If you came in, took their chocolate bars away, which one would scream the loudest? The answer is neither of them. Why? Because neither has any desire for it and if there's no desire it becomes completely irrelevant, if the person is weak-willed or strong-willed.

THE 'HOPE' METHOD

The problem is that when most people make an attempt to kick chocolate they have no strategy and have done nothing to remove their emotional hook and what is essentially their false desire. Most people simply rely on their willpower and a dash of hope to see them through. However, if a strong-willed person believes they are making a genuine sacrifice when they make the declaration 'NO MORE CHOCOLATE FOR ME' then they will be pulled in both directions and true freedom becomes a virtual impossibility. If the desire to be slim, non-spotty, healthier or whatever reason you wanted to stop for is greater than your desire for the chocolate, then they will indeed manage to 'hold out' … but for how long? After a couple of days or weeks of being disciplined, fighting a desire for chocolate and having people eating it provocatively in front of you, while teasing you with comments such as, 'Oh, this is *sooooooo* gorgeous, what a shame you can't have any, my you're doing well', most strong-willed people experience the mother of 'SOD IT' moods and completely 'crave' in – often ending up on a bit of a chocolate binge, possibly trying to make up for lost chocolate-eating time! Some people do manage to go longer, but given over 95% of the people in the UK eat chocolate, it would appear that very few actually make it to ultimate chocolate freedom.

ABSENCE WAKES THE HEART GROW FONDER

The whole willpower approach just doesn't make sense. The idea, when simplified, seems to be to reach a point where you say, 'I'VE HAD ENOUGH – THAT'S IT, NEVER AGAIN!' and then to proceed to put yourself into what can only be described as a self-imposed mental tantrum in the *hope* that if you have enough willpower to 'hang on in there' for long enough, the craving for chocolate will eventually go and you will be able to wake up one day and say to the world, 'YES, I DID IT, I'M FREE.' However, there's a slight flaw in this grand plan:

IT'S BOLLOCKS!

The willpower approach only removes the chocolate but does nothing to reverse the brainwashing or remove your desire for the stuff. I repeat: the craving for chocolate is over 95% mental, so if you only remove the physical side you are still left with a very, very big problem. You are left with the belief that you are making a huge sacrifice and missing out. You are left with the belief that you cannot enjoy or cope with parts of your life without chocolate. In other words, even though the chocolate has gone – you still have a chocolate problem! You cannot tell me that those people in Overeaters Anonymous who have been *physically* free from consuming the stuff for years, don't still have a chocolate problem. And you cannot tell me that anyone who has gone weeks or months without chocolate but are still having to use willpower not to eat it, have solved their chocolate problem in any way, shape or form. Both sets of individuals spend their time either eating the stuff and wishing they didn't, or not eating it and wishing that they could! How flipping barmy is that? So if they're eating chocolate they're not free and if they're not eating it they're not free. This is because the addiction is in the MIND! This means that even if you are without chocolate for years, if you still believe you are missing out on something worth having, then your craving will still be with you. So it appears that according to conventional thinking on chocolate addiction there only appears to be one of two options. Either eat it and suffer the mental and physical consequences of doing that or stop by using 'willpower' or 'the chocolate diet approach' and suffer the consequences of that nightmare. Either way you still suffer and still very much have a chocolate problem.

There is, of course, one other option that no one seems to have thought of – *see this 'food' for the mind-controlling, body-destroying substance that it is and jump for joy to be free at last and not to have to eat it*. Be happy about the fact you are free? What a concept – a concept which completely eluded me some years ago and one which seems to continue to elude most chocolate addicts! This is why the only option they can envisage is good old-fashioned hold your breath and hope for the best … willpower.

There were many times when I was so fed up with my chocolate eating and felt so mentally and physically shitty after eating it, that I would literally crush up and throw every last bit of chocolate in the bin with the angry declaration, 'That really is it, I mean it, NO MORE CHOCOLATE EVER AGAIN.' And I meant it, I really did! As my head hit the pillow I was convinced that 'as from *tomorrow*' chocolate was complete history. But during the night my brain seemed to turn to a mush of cocoa and the chocolate phantom had taken possession of my mind! This, of course, was mad, as I could often go days (sometimes weeks) without the stuff and it wouldn't bother me in the slightest. Yet because I had said, 'NEVER AGAIN' huge pangs of deprivation kicked in and the cravings started again. I remember managing to cope with the cravings pretty well during the day, sometimes even feeling a bit 'holier than thou' as I said, 'No thanks' to offers of chocolate. But as the night fell so the yells of 'EAT ME' came bellowing from the bin. Yes, the chocolate I had thrown away in anger the night before was all of sudden calling me and after a few, 'NO, NO, NO, I MUST BE STRONG' conversations with myself, the inevitable 'SOD IT, I COULD GET BLOWN UP TOMORROW AND CHRIST, IT'S ONLY A BIT OF CHOCOLATE – I CAN DO WHAT THE BLOODY HELL I LIKE' would rear its familiar head. This would then be followed by the even more inevitable, 'God why did I do that' which naturally was followed by the, 'Bugger it, I've started now so who cares', which was in turn followed by the declaration, 'THAT'S IT, I MEAN IT, AS FROM *TOMORROW* – NO MORE BLOOMING CHOCOLATE!' Other times I would somehow manage to go for weeks by using willpower, but I would find it pretty hard, envied everyone I saw eating the stuff and, more importantly, the *cravings* for chocolate were always there.

In fact, it appears that no matter how long you 'hang on in there' spending your life waiting for *time* to solve your chocolate problem – the craving for the chocolate *always* seems to be there to one degree or another. In many cases, as the days and weeks go by the cravings can even get worse! This proves that these cravings simply cannot be physical in any way. Even nicotine only takes two to three days to leave the system, after that it's *all* mental. With chocolate, the physical withdrawal (if you can even describe it as such), generates no physical pain and is so slight that if you blink you might miss it! But because the cravings can appear so strong

(and so they *actually are* at that time), many people are under
the terrible misapprehension that some of the craving must indeed
be physical and so out of their control. Not everyone thinks this is
enough to head to their nearest Chocoholics Anonymous meeting,
but, like Hélène, it is enough to convince them that their
'overwhelming cravings' are of a physical, rather than a mental,
nature.

CRAVE CONTROL

Because chocolate cravings seem to get worse when on the
chocolate wagon, and the willpower method is usually about as
effective as a chocolate saucepan, chocolate addicts will try just
about anything to get 'crave free'. You can now get acupuncture,
counselling, hypnotherapy, aromatherapy massage for chocolate
cravings (yes, I know!), as well as Anonymous meetings and even
something called 'crave control' patches which have the wonderful
little subheading 'Sweet Slimming Patches'. Yes, barking mad as
this may sound, you can now get skin patches to 'help reduce your
cravings for chocolate'. They are like nicotine patches in that you
stick them on your skin, but these patches don't release a steady
dose of chocolate into your bloodstream throughout the day, but
instead you stick them on your wrist and sniff them. The makers
say that if you get a chocolate craving, instead of pulling your – or
someone else's – hair out, simply have a good sniff of your patch
and all will be well. And how is smelling a patch on your wrist
meant to eliminate your cravings? Well, according to the
manufacturers:

> 'Smell is such a powerful sense that it drives our cravings for
> food. However, when we are overexposed to the aroma of foods
> we actually lose our appetite. In effect our sense of smell
> becomes overloaded or "Aromasated".'

This may be true if you're working with the stuff all day long. (I'd be very surprised if anyone who works in the Cadbury factory can stand the smell of chocolate any more.) But I don't seriously think that sniffing on a patch which smells of vanilla every now and then will do anything to overload or 'Aromasate' your senses. Now please don't try to look up the word 'Aromasated' as you won't find it. This is one of those made-up words that makers of such products come up with in order somehow to try and explain their theory. It appears the thousands of words in the *Oxford English Dictionary* aren't sufficient to try and describe how this product is meant to work, so they came up with 'Aromasated' – brilliant!

'LITTLE PATCHES OF WILLPOWER'

The manufacturers have also managed to get past the regulators and put the words 'Little Patches of Willpower' on the front of the box. But how can a patch be full of willpower? The whole 'Crave Control' idea is certainly full of something, but willpower? I don't think so. The packet states, 'After only three days you'll notice that it has helped to control your cravings!' Notice it doesn't say, 'Get rid of your cravings forever' – far from it. The patches are in a box which has a *21-day* supply – so slightly more than three days then. Does this mean once you've finished the 21-day course you are 'choc free'? NO! Nowhere on the directions does it say this is your route to chocolate freedom, it just means you have spent almost 530 for a 21-day supply of something which only claims to 'control your cravings' not eliminate them. Controlling chocolate cravings is something most people try to do a lot of the time, but instead of using a patch, they have their health, weight and skin to worry about and this normally acts as their 'little patch of willpower'. If these patches really did *stop* the craving for chocolate then you would only need one and – Hey Presto – no more cravings, but in reality they are only designed to act as a cravings *suppressant* for chocolate. This doesn't mean they will prevent another craving from rearing its ugly head in the not-too-distant future. In fact, the makers implicitly acknowledge this by supplying you with so many of them.

But at least they are meant to stop a craving in its tracks and many would say that if it helps them to say 'no' to chocolate then bring on the patches. However, not only is this a costly way to get temporarily 'crave free', but the chances of them actually preventing you from picking up a p-p-p-Penguin are, unlike the majority of people they're aimed at, pretty slim. Naturally, the makers have got scientific proof that the patches do control cravings, but I'd like to know who the blazes took part in the study. During the writing of this book I have tested these patches on several of my chocolate-addicted friends and they have all – that's 100% of them – said they didn't even remotely work. One person even had to take it off after just half an hour as the smell was making her feel sick! Maureen Young tried something similar.

'My addiction has got so bad that I have a special patch from the doctor to wear. It is supposed to stop me from craving the real thing. But so far it hasn't helped at all.'

Now there's a shocker! My conclusion is that the only way any kind of patch could possibly help you to stop eating chocolate is if you removed them from your wrist and put them over your mouth!

THE CHOCOLATE METHOD!

Now the patch sounds bizarre, especially given that even if it did work, it would only *temporarily* suppress the cravings. However, the method most people use to stop their chocolate cravings is even more bonkers, and it's one which seemingly all addicts use to stop their cravings – simply give in and have some. Yes, the most popular way to stop chocolate cravings is to eat some chocolate! No, I haven't lost it, hear me out. What I'm saying is that many people think, 'OK, even if it doesn't do anything else, at least having chocolate satisfies my craving for chocolate and stops me being a nightmare.' But once again the complete opposite holds true. Not only will it *not* stop you wanting some in the future, but it will also *increase* the craving the minute you take your first bite! This once again leaves you with a set of no-win situations. Either don't have some, try to fight a craving and feel deprived, or do indulge and battle an even larger craving not to have more or say, 'Bugger it', scoff the lot and feel like shit – what a choice!

FALSE CRAVINGS HOLD YOU PRISONER, THE TRUTH CAN SET YOU FREE

Contrary to popular belief, chocolate cravings are very, very easy to shatter, and you don't need patches, needles or a spell in a clinic to sort them out. All you need is the truth. To illustrate this clearly, imagine you are in a room and have a box of chocolates in front of you, along with what can only be described as 'the mother of all cravings'. The type of craving that would have you getting dressed to go out in a snowstorm to get a dose of chocolate type of craving; the kind that willpower stands no chance against – you know the sort. Now, with that kind of craving could anyone stop you from having one? What about if they reminded you of your weight/health/addiction problem and said it would probably be best for you not to have one, would that stop you? Somehow I think that not only would it not stop you, but a couple of black eyes might follow! However, what if you were about to reach for one and I informed you that the box of chocolates were 'experimental chocolates' and that instead of containing regular cocoa they were in fact minced rats that had been sweetened with sugar, blended with milk and other chemicals, injected with addictive substances and produced by child slaves – how much of an 'overwhelming' craving or desire would you have then? How much willpower would you need to try not to have one? And what if you're friends came in and started to dive into the chocolates, would you envy what they are doing? Would you feel deprived? Not in a million! Why? Because you no longer have a *desire* for those chocolates as you see no benefit in eating them. Once the desire is removed, so is the craving and so too is the need to exercise control or use willpower. This proves that the apparent physical compulsion is easily laid to rest once you strip the layers to reveal the truth.

Clearly chocolates aren't really made of minced rats, but they do contain theobromine, white sugar, refined fats, caffeine, a whole host of other chemicals; they do nothing genuinely to help emotions, and up to half of all mass-market chocolate has been tainted with slavery. This means that if you can expand your mind enough to see beneath every layer of this sinister chocolate wolf, you will soon start to realize that chocolate is incapable of doing anything for you. In other words, it's not that the disadvantages of eating chocolate outweigh the advantages … there are no advantages whatsoever! The only time chocolate can be seen as in any way beneficial is if you are in a situation where there is no food at all, but when was the last time you were climbing Mount Everest, living in the Third World or out in a war zone?

This is why the willpower method fails so often. The person who has made the decision to stop eating chocolate, still strongly believes the substance gives them genuine pleasure or acts as a genuine crutch. This means that at the time of stopping, although in that moment they believe the disadvantages of eating chocolate outweigh the advantages, they continue to believe that there are several advantages to eating chocolate and that they are making a sacrifice. Which is precisely why, a few hours, or days or weeks after quitting chocolate, all of a sudden the reasons why you wanted to kick chocolate in the first place go completely out of the window. This creates the mental tug-of-war again until eventually you say, 'Bugger this for a game of soldiers' and give in … *again!*

Maureen Young spent $600 on patches, 12 slimming clubs and psychotherapy to defeat her addiction but nothing worked – why? Because these did nothing to remove her mental desire for chocolate or free her of what was clearly a destructive relationship. Although chocolate was part of what was knocking her down and *creating* many insecurities, Maureen, like virtually all chocolate addicts, was under the false impression that chocolate was helping to lift her and helping to reduce the insecurities. She said she has tried to cut out chocolate in the past but gave up after suffering piercing headaches and bad tempers. This was clearly *caused* by the chocolate, but a part of her brain thought chocolate helped the very problem it was creating. The headaches were no doubt caused by the physical withdrawal, but made much worse because of the bad tempers caused by the feeling of MENTAL DEPRIVATION.

NOTHING TO FEAR BUT FEAR ITSELF

As mentioned right at the start of this book, the only reason why anyone finds it hard to release themselves from addictions of any kind is fear. The fear they will not be able to enjoy themselves the same way without the substance; the fear that life will somehow not be the same again. All drugs create *false* fear which appears real to the addict. The false emotional attachment makes them believe they are in a no-win situation. If they don't have it they feel insecure and miserable and if they do have it they hate themselves. The *truth* is the only thing which releases the fear and thus sets people truly free. Free to see it for what it is and free to choose not to have it. The FEAR Maureen, and many others around the world is suffering from is simply:

F̲ALSE E̲MOTION WHICH A̲PPEARS R̲EAL

Any insecure feeling which comes about because of releasing yourself from this drug food is a false emotion which *appears* real. The idea is to recognize it for what it is and then to enjoy literally starving the false emotion from your body and mind.

FROM THE CRADLE TO THE 'CRAVE'

The truth is that chocolate, as a substance, not only does nothing for you but it has no hold over you either. The emotional 'hook' is purely mental and can easily be removed without the need for willpower or discipline. Remember your relationship with chocolate is based on nothing but lies, deceit and fear. It's a relationship which the chocolate industry started for you at a very early age, and if they had their way, one which would be with you until the end of your days. Fortunately, breaking up is very *easy* to do; all you need is the truth and an effective mental strategy – one which will enable you to enjoy the process, not just for a couple weeks, but for life. So come with me as I …

15

Lead Us Not Into 'Temptations' – But Deliver Us From Evil!

Also lead us not into After Eights, Toblerone, Milk Tray, Mars, Celebrations and all the others including, of course, 'Temptations'! The 'deliver us from evil' may seem a bit strong, but considering that up to half of all mass-market chocolate has been tainted with slavery and also given that the ingredients in mass-market chocolate have been linked to diabetes, obesity, skin problems, the removal of a gall bladder and behavioural changes, perhaps it's not so harsh.

Luckily, leading yourself *not* into a box of temptations and finally delivering yourself from this evil is going to be one of the easiest things you've ever done. All you need to do is think outside the chocolate box, so to speak.

MOPING AROUND FOR SOMETHING WHICH WE HOPE WE WON'T HAVE

By now it should be clear that the only reason why people struggle on a 'chocolate diet', 'the recovery method' or the chocolate wagon is not because they are suffering from a genetic cocoa problem or severe withdrawal from chocolate, but simply because they feel sorry for themselves because they can no longer have something which, somewhat ironically, they hope they won't have! Now, isn't that just a touch mad? To make a decision to stop eating chocolate because it was making you fat or ill or spotty or you just hated being a slave to it, and then when you do finally kick it to start feeling sorry for yourself because you no longer have the very thing you wanted to get rid of? Isn't that just one short step away from a life in bonkersville? Isn't this the same as a child getting upset and angry because it doesn't have a toy and then if you hand it to them they say that they don't want it.

Try to imagine feeling uptight and pining away for something which you hope you won't have? Well, if you've ever been on a chocolate diet or made an attempt to kick the dark stuff using willpower you won't need to imagine – you would, as I did on numerous occasions, already have done it. And this is the main reason why everyone thinks it's hard to kick chocolate from our lives. Yet if we all just stopped the moping and the self-imposed mental tantrums and actually felt good about the fact that we now have a genuine choice and are for once in our lives totally free *not* to eat this rubbish anymore, we just might find the whole process not only easy but also enjoyable.

THE CAN'T SYNDROME

We would also find it a hell of a lot easier if we didn't tell ourselves over and over again that we can't have chocolate; in reality we can do what the heck we like, whenever we like. I used to eat chocolate most days, but as I've said, there would be times when I just didn't have any for many days and, very occasionally, weeks. Did it bother me? No! Was I using willpower in the time I had no desire for it? No! Did I suffer withdrawal? No! And I should well imagine that many of you will have also gone days or weeks without the stuff and yet it didn't bother you in the slightest. But the very second you tell yourself you can no longer have any – BOOM! – you immediately suffer from what I call – 'The CAN'T Syndrome'. The symptoms of this are feeling miserable, deprived, having mental tantrums and wanting to hurt all those who you think are conspiring to make you not have chocolate.

In order to have true freedom you need to get it clear in your mind that when you stop eating chocolate you CAN eat it whenever you wish – just as I *can* whenever I wish! The beauty is that now I can see beneath the glossy hogwash, I just *don't* wish. Non-smokers CAN, after all, smoke whenever they wish; nobody in the world is stopping them, so why don't they? Because they don't wish to! I am not your parent or teacher, you CAN do whatever you want after you have read this book – the choice is yours. But please remember why you picked it up and remember you will no longer have a choice if you do eat or drink this drug food. Drug addiction of any kind takes away the freedom of genuine choice. It must be crystal clear by now that we are not talking about a habit, a genuine pleasure, a crutch or even a genuine food – it is drug-food addiction, nothing less.

As the majority of the addiction is based on a mental hook, it goes without saying that if you tell yourself you CAN'T you will feel mentally deprived, miserable and/or go into a self-imposed tantrum. The key to freedom is: instead of saying CAN'T what we should be saying is, 'I *can* have chocolate whenever I want, but what's the point, what would it do for me?' The answer to that question is clearly – 'NOTHING'. And that's about the strength of it; there is just no point in eating it. If you eat some, it makes you feel like rubbish and you want more. Eventually, you either have to say 'NO' or carry on and stuff yourself; either way – what's the point? It doesn't make you happy, it doesn't help to relieve stress, it doesn't relieve boredom and it isn't better than sex – so what's the point? Chocolate never gives you what you *thought* it was going to and the reason for this is due to the hook being based entirely on one of the biggest illusions ever created. If you tell yourself you CAN'T have chocolate after you finish this book you are missing the whole point and setting yourself up for an unnecessary mental tantrum and ultimate failure. In fact, I have a great acronym for the word CAN'T:

CONSTANT AND NEVER-ENDING TANTRUM

And this is precisely what we put ourselves through when we keep telling ourselves we *can't* – Constant And Never-ending Tantrum. This is what those in OA are suffering from and it is also what all those on chocolate diets are suffering from. The point is you CAN stay a slave to chocolate for the rest of your life; you CAN continue feeding an industry that preys on the young and you CAN hate yourself every time you binge on the stuff. But now you have seen beneath the layers, why would you want to? The point is you can do whatever you want, whenever you want – not that you *can't*. By understanding that you always can but there's no point to it, you instantly remove the T, which is where the Tantrum (or, for some, Torture) lies. As simple as it may sound, all you need to do to find this process easy is to shift from the chocolate wagon and willpower approach, which is – 'I want, but I *can't* have' – to the correct way of thinking 'I *can*, but I don't want to have.' Or to be much more accurate, 'I can, but I don't need to, or want to anymore – I'm free!'

'THANK GOD, I'M FINALLY FREE!' is not an expression that you will ever hear from anyone on the chocolate wagon. Neither will you hear it from those on the 'recovery method' or the willpower approach. Why? Because with these approaches you can *never* be free. In fact, the 'going on a chocolate diet' approach is all about doom, gloom and misery. People hope if they suffer the 'CAN'T' misery for long enough, the cravings will eventually go, and they will reach the stage where they can say, 'YES, I'M FINALLY FREE FROM CHOCOLATE.' But as long as they still believe they have made a genuine sacrifice and retain the false belief that chocolate provides a pleasure or crutch, they can never be free. Instead, they have a feeling of complete despondency wondering *when*, not if, they will fail. Some people even count the days – as if that will somehow make it better. Addiction is the only prison I know where people count the days *after* they escape, and how long after are they going to count the days for? And given that the craving for chocolate is mental, they're going to be counting for quite some time! If the whole idea is to try to reach the stage where you can finally say, 'YES, I'M FREE', I say, why wait? Why not kick off by feeling good about your decision? Why not feel happy to be free? After all, you CAN have chocolate whenever you wish, but the reason why you have read this book is because you don't want it any more. So the choice is simple, either have it and continue hating yourself, don't have it and fool yourself into thinking you are missing out so have a tantrum, or say, 'MY GOD, I DON'T HAVE TO EAT THAT RUBBISH ANYMORE – YES, I'M FREE!'

Kicking chocolate is stupidly easy; the *only* reason why people struggle is because after they've stopped they continue to mope for something which they hope they won't have. If for whatever reason you find yourself over the first few days after you quit experiencing a 'craving' and start a silly tug-of-war in your head,

I have one simple, yet extremely effective approach to stop it in its tracks:

Either Have the Chocolate and Shut Up or
Don't Have It and Shut Up
… but whatever you do
SHUT UP!

It's only the mental tantrum which causes the problem. So either have it and shut up or don't have it and shut up, but SHUT UP! Be aware, though, that if you *do* choose to have it after you have made the jump to chocolate freedom, you won't actually be able to shut up as it's a drug food and as such it will compel you to have more. You will also have thrown away your freedom. The *only* solution is to see it for what it is, understand you CAN have it, and *jump for joy* that you are finally free from having to eat it. Remember, if you really wanted to eat chocolate and if it was so blooming wonderful you wouldn't be reading this book!

MIND YOUR LANGUAGE!

As you can see, the language we use makes the difference between making a process of change easy or difficult. This is why, as well as never saying, 'I *can't* have chocolate' and causing yourself an unnecessary tantrum, also make a point of never saying 'I've given it up' either to yourself or when people offer you some. This is what people on the chocolate wagon and willpower method do – they 'give up'. In other words, they believe something of worth has been taken from them. It's this which causes them to 'give in'. Just the expression 'I've given up' sends a signal of sacrifice to your brain. The truth is: there is absolutely nothing to give up. The sacrifices are made when you *are* addicted to chocolate. You make sacrifices to your health, your money, your self-worth and your freedom. But even if you know all this, if you keep saying, 'I've given up' over and over again your brain can be fooled into thinking you have made a sacrifice. So mind your language – you haven't 'given up' anything so don't tell yourself you have.

TWO-PRONGED ATTACK

The reason I don't eat chocolate anymore is not simply because of my weight and health, but because it does absolutely nothing for me and I hate being manipulated and controlled by anyone or anything. When I look at chocolate, I just think, 'What's the point, what will it do for me?' A very loud NOTHING always seems to hit my brain loud and clear and so I see no reason to have it. It doesn't help any of my genuine emotions, it *adds* to insecurities, it doesn't satisfy a genuine hunger and it creates false hungers – so what's the point. You are on a hiding to nothing. It's much easier to not have the stuff and be happy about it.

Another reason why I now choose to be choc-free is that I also derive no pleasure from eating something which may possibly have been produced by slaves. I once read an excellent book entitled *Fast Food Nation* and ever since then the only time I ever go into a fast-food joint is to use the toilet. Not simply because the 'food' is usually a few salt pots short of a triple heart by-pass operation, but once you have an understanding of how the companies work and how they deliberately manipulate the minds of children and adults alike, you cannot bring yourself to give them any money. I strongly believe that Eric Schlosser's excellent book created a shift in the way people look at fast-food companies and it may be what leads to McDonald's making its first loss in its history.

In the same way, I hope this book will have a similar effect with the mass-market chocolate industry. Behind their caring, happy image of the chocolate 'hero' is a world of mind manipulation and greed. For instance, they have managed to link their product to almost every public holiday. Most children now have no idea what Easter is all about, all they think is, 'Where's my chocolate egg?' And it's hard to think of the Christmas stocking now without the image coming to mind of an array of mass-market chocolate bars meshed against a piece of cardboard. Personally, even if I wasn't bothered about my own slavery to chocolate, knowing what really goes on behind the 'child-friendly advertising' and glossy packets, means that I simply cannot bring myself to eat the stuff again. And they will certainly never get another bean from me.

Cravings only come about if you feel as though you are making a genuine sacrifice or you feel you are missing out. What people really 'crave' when they turn to chocolate is an emotional 'boost' of some kind. They are craving instant happiness, or relaxation, or an end to their sugar low. But once you know that chocolate is part of the *cause* of a sugar low – and it is impossible to feed any emotion with drugs of any kind, including drug food – then you cannot 'crave it'. It's very difficult, no it's impossible, to 'crave' a substance when you know in every part of your mind and body that not only will it do nothing for you but it will also cause you to feel *worse* than you do already! It is also, I would have thought, impossible to crave something that may have been produced by child slaves and produced by companies who do whatever they can to manipulate the minds of the young to enslave them to their product for life. This is precisely what they thought they had achieved with you, until, of course, you were exposed to the truth contained within *Chocolate Busters*. The saying is:

'Fear holds you prisoner, the truth sets you free.'

If you have opened your mind and seen the truth there is now nothing that can possibly hold you back from being one of the few people on this planet who are genuinely FREE *not* to eat chocolate. So let's take all of this new-found knowledge and finally …

16

Have A Break ... And *Not* Have A Kit Kat!

One thing I have learnt about health and addiction is that everyone seems to *talk* a very good game. The amount of people I know who are always *thinking* of making a change in their lifestyle is scary. Thinking and talking about it is the same as just hoping things will happen. There is a famous saying that goes, 'the road to "some day" leads to a town called nowhere'. And nowhere is precisely where many people stay. Usually this is because they suffer from the But Syndrome – 'I would do it, *but* ... I'm having a bad time at the moment'; 'I could do it *but* ... I've got a few social occasions coming up'; 'I could do it *but* ...' – and so it goes on. People who suffer from the But Syndrome usually have a very a big one (Butt, that is!). Things like freeing yourself from chocolate addiction don't 'just happen' and won't just happen by thinking about it or talking about it. The only way to true freedom from chocolate happens when you finally stop talking and, as a famous sports company says, 'just do it'. Not in the 'not eat chocolate and *hope* you won't have any again' sense, but where you finally unhook it from your mind and *know* you will never touch it again. *Hoping* you won't have chocolate again and *knowing* you won't is the difference between 'instant' freedom and doubt, uncertainty and possible failure. It's also the difference between finding it easy or hard.

BACK TO FRONT

There is only one reason why you picked up this book and that was to bust your addiction to one of the most overused drug foods on the planet. Stripping away the layers and exposing this insidious industry for what it really is should have made your decision extremely easy. In fact, once the truth is exposed the decision is more or less made for you. Just as with the analogy of minced rats covered in cow's milk and sweetened with loads of white refined sugar masquerading as chocolate, once you know what really lies under the layers, you simply will not be able to bring yourself to touch the stuff again. I also know that if you've understood everything here, you will know that life will just be *sooooooo* much sweeter *without* chocolate.

All the time spent worrying about it; hating yourself because you've had some; going on meaningless chocolate diets; trying to cut down, exercising control and 'hoping' one day you will simply just go off it; it's all much harder than seeing it for what it is and just not having it. This is where people have it back to front. They think it's easier to continue to have chocolate than go on the chocolate wagon, and yes it is – but it's nowhere near as easy as being free of it. The mental and sometimes physical slavery to anything, no matter how slight, can never be easier than freedom. Freedom is a place where you never require willpower, discipline or self-control, or a place where you never feel like crap because you succumbed to the dark side; it's a place where you are just exactly what it says on the tin – FREE! Free to see people eating it and not envy what they're doing; free to stop for petrol without having to fuel up on mass-made chocolate at the same time; free to enjoy Easter without stuffing yourself with chocolate junkie eggs; free to take it easy *without* a Caramel; free to go out for dinner and not have to have a dessert laced with sugar and chocolate; free to make your own decisions about what *you* really want to eat; free to walk down the chocolate aisle of the supermarket without having to buy some; and free to have a break and *not* have a Kit Kat!

BREAK THE HABIT!

Freedom, as you are gathering, is not only a wonderful feeling, but it really is very easy. IT'S ONLY THE MOANING THAT MAKES IT APPEAR DIFFICULT TO KICK – if you don't mope or moan you're free the moment you say you are! However, when you have had a pattern of behaviour for many years you need to be aware that it can take a little while for your brain to adjust fully to the new way of thinking, even when it's for the better. If you have been following a certain pattern of behaviour over and over again, then that behaviour is conditioned and so a habit has been formed. There is no question that over the years your brain will have got 'habitually conditioned' to reach for chocolate as a response to certain emotions or situations. You need to understand that even though you are free from chocolate the *second* you say, 'It's over – I'm FREE!', this doesn't mean that *at times* your brain won't automatically respond in the way it has learned. This doesn't mean that you have to act on it, or that you aren't really free; it simply means your brain is in what I describe as 'the adjustment period'. The habitual ritual of, say, going to grab a chocolate bar when filling up on petrol will in all likelihood still be there for a short while. This is nothing to worry about and doesn't mean you haven't understood the book. In fact, I'd be worried if things like this didn't happen.

YOU'RE IN THE DRIVING SEAT

For years I had a car which had the immobilizer just to the right-hand side of the driver's seat. It was a simple switch that you had to press otherwise the car wouldn't start: designed, of course, to stop people stealing it. However, for insurance purposes it wasn't good enough and I had to get a different kind of immobilizer. This time it was to the left of the driver's seat and you had to put an electronic key in it to free the immobilizer and start the car. The first day I got in the car the first thing I did was to reach down the right-hand side to try and switch off the immobilizer. Clearly it had been moved and although my conscious mind was more than aware of this, my subconscious automatically went into the old pattern of behaviour. This is something you would *expect* to happen and regard as perfectly normal. For the first few days I reached for the now absent switch *every time* I went to start my car. As the week went on this became less and less until after about three weeks I had stopped doing it altogether. My point is that just because I was still going *towards* my old pattern of behaviour on and off for a few weeks, it didn't mean I was struggling with the change. Each time I realized exactly what was going on and at no point did I sit, panic and pray to God that one day I would finally adjust to my new immobilizer! My brain wasn't ever 'hoping' I would adjust, it KNEW FOR CERTAIN. When you *know for certain* then these tiny moments of adjustment pass almost unnoticed. In the same way, if you do become aware of old chocolate patterns coming forward, instead of causing doubt and dragging you down – as they could so easily have done on the chocolate wagon method – they become positive moments where you remind yourself how wonderful it is to feel free.

Similarly, I always used to travel to work along the same route five days a week. I was so 'habitually conditioned' to going that way that sometimes I would find myself halfway to work at weekends when I in fact wanted to go somewhere completely different. If you own a car this has in all probability happened to you as well. But my point is, when you realize you're on your way to work do you ever think, 'Oh well I'm halfway there now, so I might as well go in'?

NO, OF COURSE NOT. You just think, 'Bugger, that's a bit inconvenient and turn around.' A better example is perhaps when you were a kid. Do you remember getting out of bed on a Saturday and starting to get ready for school? I know I did and my brain was so *habitually conditioned* to getting up and going to school when the alarm went off that if I had accidentally set the alarm, or it was pre-set, I would naturally get out of bed and start getting ready. But what a blooming wonderful feeling when it dawned on me it was Saturday and I realized I didn't have to go in. That feeling would have been tenfold if someone had told me I'd never have to go in again. Now clearly this analogy wouldn't work for you if you loved school, but you get the picture.

The point is, although your brain and body may well go *towards* its usual pattern of chocolate behaviour even after you stop, it doesn't mean you have to go there. It also doesn't mean for one second that you have to feel miserable for not going there – in fact, just like the school situation, these can be very enlightening and almost euphoric moments. Now I do realize there are various degrees of chocolate addiction and therefore these moments will feel different for everyone. If chocolate was a *bit* of a problem for you and you weren't eating that much and didn't really binge on the stuff, then freeing yourself of this drug food may well feel good, but not as wonderful as for someone who has suffered at its hands for years. Personally, I loved the adjustment period and whenever any old patterns popped up and I realized what was going on, I had similar feelings to realizing it was Saturday! I loved going down a chocolate aisle thinking, 'You haven't got me anymore' and feeling really bloody good about it. I loved being able to say, 'No thanks' to chocolate without any struggle or feelings of deprivation at all; just a feeling of being free of it. And when I think about it, I still love it now!

TEMPTING SITUATIONS

This is why, after you quit, it is so important to put yourself in all
the same places and situations where you would normally have had
chocolate. In other words, do the complete opposite to what most
addiction specialists tell you. One of the many pieces of advice
given to addicts of any kind is 'Avoid Tempting Situations'. No
wonder people can never learn how to be free. If I wanted to adjust
to my new immobilizer, do you think I'd have had much success if I
had avoided getting my car in case I was 'tempted' to reach for the
old switch? It's the adjustment which helps the brain to learn the
new behaviour and get used to it. This clearly doesn't work that
well on the chocolate wagon as people, no matter how long they
seem to go without, still feel they're missing out and so still crave.
But when you are *mentally* free there is no need to avoid any
situation. Temptation is in the *mind* and if your mind is free of
desire you cannot be tempted no matter where you are. Think
back to the chocolate-coated minced rats. If you knew all
chocolates were made that way would you ever be 'tempted' in any
situation? NO! Would you have 'avoid' situations where people
around you were eating them in case you envied them? NO! Once
you can see something for what it is, 'cravings' and 'temptations'
can disappear in a millisecond. This is why there is no need to
avoid any situation and if your friends are going out for a meal –
GO WITH THEM!

I have always thought that giving the advice of 'avoid tempting
situations' to people who have *not* removed their desire for
chocolate is akin to asking them to stop breathing. I was 'tempted'
to eat chocolate every time I filled up with petrol, so if I took their
advice I would have to walk everywhere. 'Oh, better not go there
because if I passed a newsagent I could easily be tempted, so I'll
stay in then.' 'Oh, better not watch programme as chocolate's
always on TV.' So I guess the only option, if I took their advice,

would be to stay in with my own thoughts; so better not think of chocolate then! Which brings me to another daft suggestion these experts have when advising you on how to stop your addictions:

'*Try not to think about it*'

Of all the advice they give this is the nuttiest. It is absolutely impossible to try not to think of something. If I said to you now, try not to think about Bill Clinton, who pops into your head? Yes, Bill Clinton. You would never have thought of him unless I said 'Try not to think about him!' With this in mind, please don't worry for one second if, during your enlightening couple of weeks adjustment period, your brain isn't full of a few cups of …

17

Thinking Chocolate

Will you think about chocolate ever again? YES! Will that pose a problem? NO! Thinking about chocolate isn't the problem; it's what you think that matters. If every time you stare at the stuff, you think, 'I want some but can't have some', then you'll have problems. But if when you see it you think, 'I'm so glad I can see it for what it is. Thank God I haven't got to eat that anymore', then you'll have no problem at all.

Please be aware that during the adjustment period in particular you are bound to have old 'thought' patterns popping up every now and then. And these patterns can, unless you're careful, delude you into thinking that you are having *real* cravings for chocolate, when in fact your brain is running a 'habitual thought' as a response to a certain situation. Whenever you are feeling any kind of negative emotion or you are looking for something to give you that extra boost, your brain will hunt its data base for what it sees as a quick and easy solution. If your brain is 'habitually conditioned' to think that chocolate will somehow do the trick, it stands to reason that when you first stop – and until it fully adjusts – your brain may well ask for some chocolate in certain situations. This doesn't mean that YOU want it, in much the same way that I didn't actually want to drive to work on my day off; it just means your brain is in a period of adjustment. Sometimes all you will hear in your head is, 'I want some chocolate.' Now unless you know what's really happening, it can be very easy for you to think that this is a *genuine* craving. Remember, though, if you really loved chocolate so much and life was always so sweet with it, then you wouldn't be reading this book and you wouldn't want to be free of it. So if you ever get the thought, 'I want some chocolate' you need to understand it's not YOU who wants it – it's simply an old thought pattern and this doesn't mean 'IT' is not working.

This is something I used to get at my clinic, The Vale Centre. Whether a client had come for help with stopping smoking, quitting alcohol or getting off drug foods such as mass-market chocolate, if they ever had thoughts of, 'I want a …' (whatever the old pattern addiction was for them), they would inevitably start to blame me or more accurately – 'IT'. They would phone up and say (sometimes rather loudly), 'IT'S NOT WORKING' or 'IT HASN'T WORKED.' But one thing you must understand if you are to have lifelong freedom – there is no IT. IT is YOU, and if YOU have opened up your mind enough to see this hyped-up drug food for what it really is and if you follow my guidelines (a simplified breakdown of which are at the end of the book, *see* Chapter 20) you will find that 'IT' works! If YOU don't open up then IT won't work. I will repeat it one more time:

'IT' IS YOU!

I have had many thousands of e-mails from people who have freed themselves of the whole 'food trap' using the information contained within my first bestselling book, *Freedom from the Diet Trap: Slim for Life*, but I've also heard a few people say, 'The book didn't work'. What is crazy is that they actually think it is down to the book. The expression 'You can lead a horse to water …' springs to mind. I can only show you the way. I can only expose the industry for what it is and hope you are brave enough to let go mentally and enjoy your new-found choc-free lifestyle. If you go back to your chocolate 'addiction' after you have read this book, it doesn't mean the BOOK didn't work – it means YOU have failed to act on the information in the book. The only difference between those who succeed in life and those who fail is that the former act on information and the latter talk about acting on information. My aim here is to make sure not only that IT works, but also to make the IT as easy as possible. The truth is, IT is easy; it is only *you* who can make the process difficult by sitting and moping for something which you hope you won't have! Remember the hard part is being a slave to this drug food, the easy part is your jump to freedom. I just want to make sure that you don't misinterpret any 'thoughts' you may have for chocolate, not just in the first couple of weeks, but throughout your life.

During the first few weeks is when most of the old thought patterns will manifest themselves, but if you understand why they are there, then you won't start thinking 'IT'S NOT WORKING.' By interrupting the old pattern of thought and not giving it any power – IT will be working every time. So all you need to do if a 'thought' pops in your head such as 'I want some chocolate' or 'Wouldn't that be nice' is to see it for what it is – just a thought. A thought triggered by an old way of responding to certain situations or feelings. It doesn't mean the thoughts are genuine ones and it doesn't mean you have to act on them. After all, do we act on all our thoughts? NO, if we did we'd probably be arrested! Thoughts only contain the power YOU give them. If you don't feed the thought, it will die *immediately* and you will feel completely free before you know it.

FOOD FOR THOUGHT

This is why it is essential that if or when these old thought patterns pop up from time to time, you don't feed them with insecurity, panic or moaning! This is the only reason why people find it hard: they feed the thought instead of destroying the thought. This is why it is pointless to try to think of something else or try to keep yourself busy. It is very important to *acknowledge* the thought, understand why it's there, see it for the powerless thing it really is and enjoy *not* having to feed it. If you try to 'take your mind off it' you will lose the ability to adjust, the thought will grow until it has the potential to turn into a real craving, and then 'IT' may not work. This is why people fail so often when they try to quit without any mental preparation. Every time an old pattern of thought pops up they feed into it and sit around *hoping* it will go away. But you and I know that if someone's nagging at you and you ignore them, they start to shout louder! These old patterns of thought can do the same unless you know what you're doing. Luckily, you do know what you're doing and you are also armed with the truth about chocolate; this combination means *chocolate doesn't stand a chance*. When any thought of chocolate rears its head, you will now understand why it's there and immediately destroy it by saying, 'I used to have to act on this, but now I don't have to – YES, I'M FREE!' I know this may seem over the top to some of you as everyone's degree of addiction to chocolate is slightly different, but I must say whether you expect it or not, when you are in situations where you simply don't want chocolate – you'll feel bloody good! You will feel even better when you see others around you tucking in. Talking of which, please understand that although you may well be pretty chuffed at becoming one of the very few people in this country who are free from mass-market chocolate, others around you may not share in your new-found choccie freedom. You may well have your thoughts licked, but to make sure of your success, never underestimate the power of …

18

Chocolate Addicts Everywhere

As we have seen, chocolate is a pretty emotive subject and chocolate addicts everywhere will not simply accept that you don't want it anymore. Over the next few weeks you will find that chocolate is one of the few drug-like substances on this planet which you have to justify *not* taking. If you turn it down, people will assume you are either on a diet, on the chocolate wagon or have gone barking mad. What they find almost impossible to get their head round is that you just don't want the stuff anymore. Such is the power of chocolate conditioning that the concept is almost alien to everyone.

IT'S THE DRUG FOOD TALKING

One thing I learnt very quickly when I freed myself is that people don't mind you not eating drug foods like chocolate … *providing you're miserable about it!* If you are happy, not moaning, not moping but actually loving it, they hate you. Hate is perhaps too strong a word, but they certainly don't like it one little bit. The truth and irony is that they will actually be jealous of you and envy you for not having it. This is why the chocolate wagon is so nuts. You have the people on the wagon envying the people who are eating chocolate and those who have eaten chocolate envying the ones who are on the wagon! How nuts is that? Every time I have some juicy strawberries I never wish I hadn't had them and I don't envy the people who turn them down – I just think: 'You don't know what you're missing.' Yet as soon as people finish a load of chocolate they always say out loud (or think), 'Oh bugger, I wish I hadn't had that' and nine times out of ten they envy those who skipped the stuff. When I see other people eating chocolate I never envy their situation; I actually look and think: 'What a shame, if only you knew.' So be aware that no matter what they say, no matter how aggressive or Mickey-taking they are, please understand it's not them – it's just the drug food talking!

Nobody likes to take their drug alone, and I don't mean alone as in 'by themselves', I mean alone in company. If you are at a meal with a couple of friends and they want a piece of Death By Chocolate, be aware that a simple 'no thanks' won't suffice; if you're on a diet and say, 'God, I'd love some but I'm on this diet and, you know, I'm only allowed X points a day and that will go way past my quota' then they'd leave it at that. It may prick their conscience and they may well wish (afterwards) that they hadn't had it, but as long as they think *you* are having a bad time – they'll be as happy as a mouse on a trip to Edam. In fact, you'll often find them making all kinds of noises as they eat it and will say stuff like, 'Oh, this is *sooooooo* good, what a shame you can't have any.' But if you say, 'I can have some, nothing's stopping me, I just, don't want any', they won't leave it at that. Not having any *and* feeling good about it (a unique concept) instantly makes them aware of what they're doing and so they feel the need to justify their chocolate eating – 'Oh, you only live once, anything could happen tomorrow' or 'I'm going on a diet on Monday [when else!] so I'm allowed' or 'I don't put on weight so I can get away with it.'

The actress Hélène Mahieu is as thin as a rake, but she doesn't 'get away with it' – 'IT' being a mental and physical slave to a drug food and 'Derren Browned' on a massive scale by an unscrupulous industry. Just because someone doesn't suffer the symptoms of overweight with this drug food, doesn't mean they 'get away with it'. There are many people whose addiction to chocolate is so strong that virtually all they eat is chocolate. The reason they don't gain weight is because they are 'controlling' their intake and having little bits throughout the day and *nothing else*. But no matter what excuse people come out with you can be certain they are only voicing it because they would actually love to be in a position where they didn't want it – like you. This is why as you sit there perfectly happily, seeds of envy are sprouting in their minds. As they choose the dessert *and* while they are eating it, you will hear comments either of justification or attacks on you and your personality. 'Go on, won't you join us?' 'What's the matter with you, you boring sod' and so it goes on. But the only reason why they are making such a big meal of it is that by not 'needing' any, you have shown them that they do. So all I'm saying is, watch out for other people eating chocolate around you, not because by seeing them you will get tempted, but because they will resort to all kinds of power of persuasion to make sure you 'join them' again. Again, please remember it's not really them – it's just the drug food talking.

There are, of course, those people who have the odd bit of chocolate and it really isn't much of a problem for them (yes, they do exist!) but these people are much rarer than you think, and even they find the reality nothing like they expected. You won't be able to spot the genuine take-it or leave-it chocolate eaters since all drug addicts lie, including drug food addicts, but trust me they are rare and if they loved it so much they would have it more often.

INVASION OF THE BODY SNATCHERS

Any industry which manipulates the minds of children, regardless of how they damage their health, simply in order to gain profits by emotionally hooking them, will not get my money and I will never be part of their game again. I even refuse to buy chocolate for the children who are part of my life. The last thing I want to be is part of the problem. Of course, it is easier to give already addicted children some chocolate, not simply so you won't get abuse from them, but also from their parents. However, what is easiest is not always what is right. I find that the parents are the real obstacle as they think you are being mean, and again the old 'it's only a bit of chocolate' mantra gets spouted at you. But anyone can go on the Internet and send someone some chocolates; personally I prefer to make the effort to be there and play with them. A children's birthday party shouldn't be about how much drug food is on offer, but what games can be played and what stories told. For my goddaughter's 6th birthday party I spent time getting together a small basket of the finest fruits for her. I'm not saying this to boast, 'Oh, aren't I good' but simply to illustrate that the pressure out there, not just from the industry itself, but from the people who have already been conditioned is frightening. It's like invasion of the chocolate snatchers, as if they've all been possessed, and in a way they have! The industry spends so much money on advertising, yet once they've got people under their chocolate spell, it appears there's little need. The chocolate addicts will do all the pressure selling for them. Clearly, it's your call whether you choose to buy chocolate for other people when you stop, but when it comes to children at least, it's worth being different.

CHOCOLATE SUBSTITUTES

Whatever you do, don't make the fatal error of looking to 'replace' chocolate with some kind of chocolate alternative, such as carob. This is for two reasons. One is that you need to remember what you are doing is breaking an emotional attachment and a pattern of behaviour. If you reach for an alternative during times when you would have usually had chocolate then you have missed the whole point. The idea of breaking free is to be free of reaching for *any* drug food as a response to emotion. Having more of a different drug food at these times doesn't remove the problem at all – it just moves it. The second reason is that chocolate alternatives like carob are often just as bad on the health front as the real thing – and in some cases even worse. Carob in particular has always had a 'healthy' image and is to be found in all 'good' health shops. However, whereas *some* chocolate is free of hydrogenated vegetable oil, carob is loaded with the stuff. It is also packed with the cocaine of the food world – sugar! The only time when carob is OK is when you buy carob powder. It is then free of sugar and hydrogenated oil, and as long as you are not using it to try to change an emotion, you're in no danger of carob powder hooking you back onto the real thing. The only time I ever use carob powder, and even then very rarely, is when I add it to a fruit smoothie when a bunch of kids pop round. This is not because I want to get them into anything which resembles chocolate, but more because they are already on the stuff and I can offer a healthier alternative.

Some people stop eating chocolate and replace it with other high-sugared alternatives. But getting rid of chocolate and replacing it with 'sugar sweets' is like coming off cocaine and going on to speed! I don't know if you will take the information in this book and use it for *all* high-sugar sweets (I sincerely hope you do), but if truth be told, if you just skip anything containing chocolate it will certainly help to give this industry the much needed licking it deserves. However, if you do reach for carob and other sweets as some kind of replacement, you will send the wrong signals to your brain which will give it the false impression that you have made a sacrifice. Reaching for a substitute for chocolate is like a cigarette smoker taking up a pipe! Nicotine is nicotine no matter what vehicle is used to drive it into the bloodstream and white refined junkie sugar is white refined junkie sugar no matter what it's encased in.

YOU HEALTH FREAK!

The only substitute you need to make is from bad health to good, and getting rid of mass-market chocolate (and other high-sugared confectioneries) will certainly help in that area. I am aware that the majority of people who read this book will have some kind of challenge with their health – even if, unlike Maureen Young, they can't visibly see it. Often people can look OK on the outside but they are slowly breaking up from within. This is why you sometimes hear of fit-looking people who die playing tennis at the age of 40! They looked fine, but their blood vessels and organs were slowly getting clogged. There is no question that years of chocolate/sugar addiction will have left their mark. For some, the 'mark' is very obvious and they have been left with the ultimate chocolate/sugar hangover. I'm not talking here about the headaches which can come about as a direct result of caffeine and theobromine withdrawal, but about the hangover from which over half the population of the UK suffers – 'The Flesh Hangover'! We are now in a situation where over half the population of the UK is overweight or clinically obese, so many people reading this book will fall into this category due to their addiction. For others the 'mark' is not in the form of overweight, but bad skin, dull eyes and lack of energy. For others, the 'mark' is not so obvious. But no matter what category you fall into, if you have been eating mass-market chocolate and high-sugared sweets and biscuits for years, it will have left a mark somewhere.

The good news is that getting rid of chocolate from your life and stopping eating all drug-like sugary foods in response to emotions, will certainly go a long way in removing these marks. What will help catapult you even faster to the land of the slim, trim and healthy is to make a small investment which will take your health to a whole new level. Get a juicer! Juicing is simply the fastest way to get raw 'live' nutrients into your clogged and starving cells. Juices not only feed the body what it needs to repair and thrive but also flush the system of waste (like excess fat!). I do not have time to go into this subject here – this book's about chocolate – but I imagine you would not have picked up this book if you weren't interested in your *overall* health. (For more on this, get hold of *The Juice Master's Ultimate Fast Food*, or visit **www. thejuicemaster.com**)

When you stop eating drug foods like chocolate and start to furnish your body with live produce in the form of juice and whole fruits, something truly incredible starts to happen. Your eyes get brighter, your hair starts to shine, your skin glows, you lose weight (if your body needs to), your nails get stronger, your breathing gets easier, your head feels clearer, your thinking is sharper, and your energy levels explode! But again, please watch out. When you make the change from bad health to good, not everyone will be as pleased as you. Remember, people eating rubbish get upset if you stop eating chocolate and are happy about it, and that's without any physical improvements taking place. Trust me, once they see you losing weight, looking amazing and having more energy, they will not be best pleased. Once again, this isn't because it's in their nature to be mean and nasty, but if they feel they can't pull themselves out of where they are, the natural tendency is to try to drag you down. This is why they'll say things like, 'You used to be fun', 'You've changed', 'You're not the same anymore' and the most common one of all – when the physical changes really start to kick in – 'You health freak.' Chocolate addicts everywhere will seemingly do anything and say anything to try to lure you back – so always be on your chocolate guard!

Well, that's almost it, but before you depart into your new choc-free world, I have one final and very important warning. Many

people, when exposed to the truth, do manage to become free –
but how many manage to stay free for life? With the information in
this book, you would think everyone; however – and this is perhaps
the most frustrating part for me – some people understand
everything in the book, believe everything and follow everything …
except this final guideline. Unless you get your head round this last
chapter the chances are your mind will shift back and you'll be
back on the chocolate before you know it. The need for others to
have you 'join them' can be pretty strong and they will spend many
hours over the next few years trying to convince you that, 'Oh,
come on, it's only chocolate, it's not like we're talking cigarettes
here is it? Just one won't hurt.' If this is said enough and it has
been a while since you kicked the chocolate, you could start to
believe it yourself. However, what you need to realize is that one
will hurt because …

19

One Nibble And You're Nobbled!

The makers of the chocolate chip cookies Hob Nobs are the first to point out that 'One Nibble and You're Nobbled' and if you want to make sure you never get suckered back in, their advice is certainly worth listening to.

No matter how long you have stopped for, if you decide to make just *one* situation 'different' and get fooled into thinking 'one won't hurt' – BOOM – you'll be back in the hands of the chocolate industry before you can say 'Nobbled'. The reason for this is *not* because chocolate has such a powerful physical addiction but because if you believe that 'one' will somehow change or enhance your emotional state, you will think a million will do the same. So you may only have the 'one' that day or night and you may well not crave any the next day or the next week. But this doesn't mean the seeds of doubt have not already been sown. Your brain is then fooled into a false sense of security and in turn you are fooled into thinking that by not having any cravings for chocolate for the ensuing days or weeks this proves that chocolate can never be a problem for you again. You then find yourself in a situation where chocolates are being passed around again and now you falsely think, 'I know one won't hurt, I proved that last week.' Before you know it the 'one' which can't hurt has turned into 50 and you are back trying to control your intake like everyone else. For some the slow part of this process doesn't happen at all, as soon as they have one – WHAM! – they instantly go on an almighty binge. But whether it's instant or drawn out, the end result is inevitable – hooked again! I want to make it clear that if someone force-fed you chocolate or it was in something which you thought was choc free, you wouldn't get hooked. You would only get hooked if you reached for it yourself believing that you would gain something by eating it. I cannot stress enough that the 'hook' is virtually all psychological. I could eat ten large bars of the stuff in front of you now but I couldn't get hooked. I could only get hooked if I reached for chocolate believing there was some kind of genuine pleasure or crutch to be gained by eating it. If you asked me to eat some to prove I wasn't hooked I could easily do it – it wouldn't be me wanting it, I'd merely be making a point.

There will never be a need for you 'to make a point' so don't even think about it. Once you are free, enjoy it and if any moments of doubt rear their ugly heads in the future, remind yourself of why you read this book in the first place. As far as I'm concerned there is only one occasion where eating chocolate is more than justified and where you wouldn't get hooked if you did – when your lover has melted some over their naked body and asks you to lick it off! (Thank heavens there are exceptions to every rule!) The reason why, if you licked the chocolate, you *wouldn't* get hooked is because it's not the chocolate you want – it's the … well, you know. But other than that, if you make the exception to have 'just the one' you will be nobbled! If people could have just the *one*, then this book would never have come about and the chocolate industry wouldn't be turning over billions. It is true that just one chocolate never hurt anyone, but then neither did *one* cigarette. It's the drug-like chain reaction which causes the problem and one leads to the next and the next and the next … If you make one exception you will make a million. And don't be fooled for one second into thinking that if you did have *one* and you did get hooked again, it wouldn't reach a 'million exceptions' because you could simply read this book again and be free. Let me make this point very clear, so you never even begin to think it.

THE BOOK IS NEVER THE SAME TWICE!

If there is any danger with the methodology in this book, it is that it makes it easy to kick chocolate. How can that be a danger, I hear you ask? People who find it easy to stop can always find it easy to start again. This is a category you do not want to fall in as this book will not have the same impact a second time around. The reason for this, if I didn't make it clear enough a second ago:

THE BOOK IS NEVER THE SAME TWICE!

The information in this book is new to you at this moment. What I mean is, it's fresh and has been presented in such a way that your brain should respond by saying, 'Ah, I have never seen it that way before; that way of thinking makes so much sense.' This book is designed to expose the drug-food mass-market chocolate industry for what it is and give you a unique way of thinking which will make the process of freeing yourself easy and enjoyable. If you were ever to get caught in the trap again and tried to reread the book, the information and the way in which it is presented would no longer be fresh. You would find yourself skipping pages and saying, 'Yeah, I know that, I know that.' You would then reach the end and say the book doesn't work anymore. But the book never changes, only the way in which the person reading it perceives it.

USE YOUR SIXTH SENSE TO REMAIN FREE

Have you seen the film *The Sixth Sense* starring Bruce Willis? If not, I won't spoil the ending, but you get the point. If you have seen it I doubt if you knew what was going to happen at the end. This film has a slow beginning but a great twist at the end. However, if you have seen the film and tried to get the same impact by watching it again, you could never manage it, no matter how hard you tried. All that happens to those who do watch it again is that they just sit there analysing the film.

Exactly the same applies to this book. But why would you ever want to read it again? It is designed for people who are addicted to chocolate; you no longer fall into that category and if YOU have anything to do with it you never will. You picked up this book and have read this far because you were either consciously or subconsciously looking for a way to kick the chocolate. You have found one – so use it. Once free it would be nuts to go back EVER, especially when you know that it's all one huge mind-controlling illusion and that the chances of an easy and enjoyable escape a second time around are virtually nil! Keep the book by all means – in fact, I urge you to do so. You can use the information contained within as a great re-tuning tool – but not as a 'get out of chocolate jail free card'. The brainwashing and conditioning for this drug food are second to none, so it's good to go back over certain chapters from time to time. Never underestimate the power of chocolate pressure and brainwashing; to remind you one last time, the chances are if you do have just *one* nibble you'll be:

WELL AND TRULY NOBBLED!

You are now armed with the information and a way of thinking which, if followed, makes the process of busting your chocolate 'addiction' easier than probably anything you've ever done. To make life even easier and to be sure that you don't forget any of the key points over the adjustment period, here are …

20

The Guidelines

THE DECISION

Once you have made the decision to be choc free, never doubt your decision. Doubting is like 'thought cancer' and can spread rapidly. *Knowing*, not *hoping* that you have made the right decision will kill doubt instantly. You have clearly made the right decision, so don't drive yourself mad by questioning whether it's the right one. Remember, if you didn't want to kick the chocolate you would never have picked up this book. If doubt ever starts to rear its ugly head, be safe in the knowledge that it's just an old pattern being triggered by a certain emotion or situation and it has no power other than the power YOU give it. You are not only making a decision not to have chocolate for health/weight reasons, but also for slavery reasons. And I'm not simply talking about your mental and physical slavery to this drug food, but the child slavery which often goes into producing the stuff. So, for your and their sake, never doubt your decision.

THERE IS NOTHING TO GIVE UP

Your brain is an extraordinary computer, but whatever you program in, it will believe – even if it's not true. This is why *what* you say to yourself after you've made the decision is so important. If every time someone offers you some chocolate you say, 'No thanks, I've given it up' your brain can easily start to believe it has made a sacrifice. Just the expression 'given up' implies a sacrifice. This is why, small point though it may seem, you should never use the expression 'I've given up.' Not because you are trying to trick your brain, but because you genuinely haven't *given up* anything worth having. All the emotional and situation 'boosting' abilities of chocolate are just one huge illusion. The fact is you're not 'giving up' anything – you are *getting rid* of one of the biggest drug foods from your diet. This is the difference between your brain *thinking* it's made a sacrifice and *knowing* it hasn't, and it is the difference between success and failure. The only reason why people struggle when on the chocolate wagon is because they believe they have 'given up' – so now you know you haven't, don't start telling your brain you have by using the expression 'I've given up.' Instead use expressions like, 'I've kicked it', 'I don't need it anymore' or 'I've got rid of that from my life' – you get the idea!

NEVER SAY I CAN'T

Constant **A**nd **N**ever-ending **T**antrum is all you can expect to achieve if you start telling yourself you *can't* have chocolate. You *can* have chocolate whenever you like, no one is stopping you. But now you understand the nature of the beast, why would you want to? The fact is, you don't want to anymore, so don't drive yourself cuckoo by using the word 'can't'. Remove the 'T' from the word and you have immediately removed the self-imposed tantrum.

THERE IS NO SUCH THING AS A CHOCOHOLIC

I know this doesn't apply to everyone reading this book, but your chocolate addiction was never due to the fact you were any kind of 'olic'. One of the biggest mistakes most addiction experts make is that they believe it is the person rather than the substance that is the problem. Once again, since everyone who jumps in quicksand sinks, nobody in their right mind should ever blame the person. The mistake is made because the rate at which everyone sinks is always slightly different. Most people are sinking so slowly that they aren't aware they're sinking at all. Those who sink slightly faster than others or who are aware that they are sinking, are given labels such as '-olic' and are banished to a life of 'recovery'.

If you are 'in recovery' for the rest of your life you can never recover! But how long does it take to recover from chocolate addiction? There are hardly any painful physical withdrawal symptoms to contend with, and even if there were they would be gone in a few days. The fact is that nobody is pre-disposed to chocolate addiction and no one is a chocoholic. Chocolate addiction is only due to a clever emotional hook created by slight physical false hungers and backed up by false advertising. If you thought you were ever a chocoholic, let go – you're not!

THINKING CHOCOLATE

Don't try *not* to think about chocolate or worry about it if you are thinking about it a lot of the time. If I had just read an entire book on tennis, then there is no question I would be thinking about it a lot more than I usually do. Expect to think about chocolate – it would be pretty weird if you didn't just after making the decision to quit. Make sure that whenever you do think about it, whether it's today, tomorrow, next week or for the rest of your life – that you also think, 'Thank God I don't have to eat that rubbish any more; thank goodness I'm free of it.' That way you can think about chocolate every minute of the day and you will still be happy. It is *what* you think that makes the difference.

DON'T MOAN – REJOICE!

This is a key guideline. Remember there is nothing to moan about. You are not making a genuine sacrifice, you're not going to suffer a painful withdrawal and you're doing what *you want* to do. How pathetic and pointless would it be to spend any amount of time feeling sorry for yourself because you no longer have something you don't want! One of the most insane things seemingly intelligent people do is to spend time moping around for something which they hope they won't have. Enjoy your freedom from the start and rejoice never having to be part of the chocolate industry's mind-manipulation games ever again.

DON'T COUNT DAYS

Again this is where so many people go wrong. They start counting the days since they stopped as if 'time' will somehow solve their problem. Are they going to count days for the rest of their lives? What are they waiting for? The day when they can say, 'I'm free'? If they sit around moaning and counting days they will *never* be able to say it. If someone lifted you out of quicksand, would you start counting the days since you were out? NO! You would simply be glad to be out and then get on with your life. Do the same with regards to mass-market chocolate and freedom will be felt instantly.

DON'T AVOID *ANY* SITUATIONS

This guideline is self-explanatory – you have stopped eating chocolate you have not stopped living!

NEVER LOOK BACK WITH 'ROSES'-COLOURED GLASSES

The grass is not greener on the other side, if it were you would never have wanted to stop in the first place. This reminds me of people who spend ages plucking up enough courage finally to get out of a painful relationship only to meet their ex for coffee a few weeks or months later. Before they know where they are, the other person has moved back in and once again they are fearful of letting go – it can be years, if at all, before they pluck up the courage again. Time, it seems, can lead to a touch of amnesia! With this in mind, understand that as time goes by your brain can easily be fooled into thinking that meeting chocolate just 'once' for coffee won't do any harm. But – one nibble and you will be nobbled!

DON'T ENVY CHOCOLATE EATERS – PITY THEM!

This is perhaps one of the single most important guidelines of them all. When you see anyone eating or drinking chocolate never envy what they are doing. If you have fully understood the information in this book you will know there is nothing to envy and everything to pity. The truth is everyone who eats chocolate in front of you will actually be envying you. This is because the *reality* of eating chocolate never matches the *anticipation*. This is because the anticipation of what you think you'll be getting is based on millions of Derren Brown mind and taste manipulation moments.

THIS BOOK IS NEVER THE SAME TWICE!

That's about the fourth time I've written that sentence in this book and for good reason. Never treat this book as some kind of safety net; it will not be the same second time around.

AND FINALLY, follow these guidelines and pretty soon you will experience …

21

The 'Ripple' Effect

Chocolate is a highly emotive subject. Whenever it is a topic (pun intended) on a TV or radio phone-in, you can be sure the phone lines will light up. When it's on the front cover of a magazine, it sometimes has a better effect on sales than the picture of a Hollywood star! Everyone and their mother have an opinion on chocolate and given the chance they will want to share it. So please fully expect to get embroiled in many long discussions when you mention either *Chocolate Busters* or your decision to kick chocolate. What you will find is that once people realize you are serious, have no earthly intention of ever going back and are using expressions like, 'I'm free of that stuff' or 'I don't need it any more', you will start to witness 'The Ripple Effect'.

On the surface, of course, people will argue their chocolate corner and will say things like, 'You've been brainwashed, it's only a bit of bloody chocolate, you nutter' or 'I don't have a problem with chocolate and I've got no intention of ever stopping.' However, you will notice that as time goes on your freedom will become contagious to even the hardiest of chocolate 'lovers'. They won't make a huge song and dance about it, but you can expect them to ask discreetly, 'What was the title of that book again?' Naturally, they will say it's for someone else, that they're just curious, or they want to hear more about the slavery in chocolate, but *most* people will become more than curious.

I for one really hope they do. Gone are the innocent days when people like John Cadbury and Milton Hershey had a dream and genuinely thought that chocolate was good for you. These were good men who provided not only the finest working conditions, but set up whole communities with a much higher standard of living than most. When I talk of chocolate and mind manipulation I'm not talking of these good people; I'm talking about the greed at any health cost which has plagued the chocolate industry for years. I'm talking about people who know full well how their product and advertising can entice and hook children. People who know that the ingredients, if eaten in quantity and over a long period of time can (like cigarettes) cause great harm to health. Not all chocolate firms are tarnished with the same brush. There are quite a few little shops still producing what they see as good chocolate – chocolate which has as little sugar and as much cocoa as possible; chocolate with a Fair Trade label attached. These people clearly mean no harm and anyway high-cocoa chocolate is pretty difficult to get addicted to. It is the mass-market high sugar version ones which the book focuses on.

The mass-market chocolate industry has had a goody-two-shoes image for far too long. There was a blip in the early 1970s when Michael Jacobson coined the phrase 'junk food' and included chocolate within the category. But in recent years, especially since the late 1990s, chocolate has somehow achieved an 'it's good for you' and 'a little of what you fancy does you good' image. It's also got a 'family friend' persona. This reminds me of when you see someone acting like butter wouldn't melt in their mouth, but behind closed doors their awful true colours are exposed. The idea behind writing this book was to show fully the true colours of the chocolate industry, not the ones they wish to portray. The idea was, and is, to change not just yours, but the whole world's perception of this 'wouldn't hurt a fly, aren't we good to kids' industry.

One in five children under four-years old is overweight, one in ten is classed as obese and over half of *all* people in the UK are considered to have an overweight disorder of some kind. Obesity has risen faster in Britain than anywhere else in Western Europe and diabetes is now getting out of all proportion. Mass-market chocolate is certainly playing its part in these ever-increasing numbers. Yet despite this they still have the audacity to often promote their product as 'healthy' and claim they are helping to reduce weight and health problems. When Kraft, who make Toblerone, Terry's All Gold, Terry's Chocolate Orange and products such as Dairylea, announced that they were going to be removing hydrogenated oils (trans-fatty acids) from their 'foods', they had the front to say,

> 'The rise in obesity is a complex public health challenge of global proportions. It can be solved only if all sectors of society do their part.'

Are they kidding? Do they honestly believe that getting headlines in newspapers about how they are 're-writing their recipes for the health of the nation' will fool us into thinking they are not part of the cause? The only reason why companies like Kraft and Master Foods (Mars) decided to remove trans-fatty acids from *some* of their products was simply a pre-emptive move so they didn't get sued. Philip Morris has already been bitten once with lawsuits from its tobacco business, the last thing they need is a fall in share price in their chocolate interests due to more lawsuits. Henry Anhalt, director of Kids Weight Down, an obesity programme based in New York warned of 'Large law-suits, class action suits looking at cardiovascular disease, premature death and diabetes'.

I was the first person to make the distinction between 'normal' food and drug food. Luckily my message seems to be getting out and more and more people are becoming wise to it. At the time of writing there are many people taking fast-food companies to court, claiming their 'foods' are addictive. The chocolate companies have escaped so far and by grabbing headlines with news of 'helping the nation's health' they are doing their best to make sure it stays that way. They will claim that 'as soon as we found out about them we removed the heart disease causing fats', but any oils they replace these with will still be refined and will still be a long way from healthy. It has taken years for trans-fatty acids to get bad press; before that they had passed 'All Government Approval'. The tobacco companies knew as far back as the early 1970s just how addictive and bad *their* product was, but in the name of profit decided to be economical with the truth. The chocolate gang are doing the same with their product. But even if the new fats are slightly better, they still won't be 'good fats' and the mass-market chocolates will remain full of white refined sugar – the major cause of obesity and diabetes.

This is why the whole 'Cadbury Get Active' campaign was a complete piss take. How dare a mass-market chocolate company say they are doing it to *help* prevent obesity and improve health? *Food Magazine* reported that a 10-year-old would have to eat so many bars to earn a basketball with their 'tokens' that it would take 900 hours of playing basketball to try and burn off the calories! And if a school wanted a new volleyball net the children would have to get through a whopping 5,440 chocolate bars! We can't even rely on the people elected to help protect our children's health from the drug-food global players, since, as we have seen, Labour sports minister, Richard Caborn, endorsed the campaign.

All of this explains why the 'ripple effect' is so important; why it is so important that people get hold of the truth so they can make an educated choice about chocolate. By opening your mind, seeing beneath the cleverly disguised layers covering the chocolate wolf, and having the courage finally to end your relationship with the stuff you will help many people do the same. The sight of you enjoying *not* having to eat the drug-food chocolate will slowly but surely send ripples of admiration and curiosity through other people's minds. Their curiosity will eventually get the better of them and in the end they will either think, 'Well, if they can do it so can I', use their willpower, but still succeed in the end, or they will buy this book, realize the truth and take the easy leap to chocolate freedom. I can guarantee that every time someone eats chocolate in front of you and you happily decline to, you will prick their conscience and curiosity, and the ripple effect will have begun. You will also find that if you have chosen to use this book as a catalyst to improve other areas of your diet and health and have decided to 'get juiced', people will soon want to know what you are doing. When the weight starts to come off (if you need to lose weight), as your eyes become brighter and as your skin starts to glow – everyone will want a piece of it. This is when 'the ripple effect' really starts to kick in. Instead of chocolate addicts dragging you back in, just by being free and getting juiced you will help to lift them out.

Unlike some I have a *genuine* passion for what I do. At The Vale Centre in England, I have run sessions for weight loss/health, stopping smoking, quitting alcohol, and even for chocolate addiction for years. But if I saw everyone on an individual basis it would take thousands of years to get this message out. That's why I wrote *Freedom from the Diet Trap: Slim for Life* – there is no way I could have physically seen each and every one of the people who have had their lives changed with that book if I had seen them individually. And we can speed up the rate at which the world hears the truth about mass-market chocolate – by telling everyone we meet to get the book! I know this sounds like a bit of an ad, but the only reason why I wrote *Chocolate Busters* was to get the information to as many people as I can in the quickest possible time.

I genuinely want this book to have a *Fast Food Nation* effect on the chocolate industry and that will only happen by people reading it, freeing themselves and telling others. Everybody doesn't need to buy the book; they can get it from the library – I really don't care! I just want people to see this stuff for what it is and help turn the tide. With your freedom and help, the 'ripple' will soon turn into a tidal wave and the chocolate industry won't know what's hit them. *Chocolate Busters* is designed to do exactly what it says on the tin – bust the industry and bust your addiction.

Thank you for taking the time to read this book. I sincerely hope that if nothing else it has helped you to kick the chocolate … *and be happy about it!* I love to hear from people who have made changes to their life after reading my books, so please, if you get the time, send me an e-mail or drop me a line. Unless I'm up to my ears in it, I try to make a point of reading and replying to all my mail. If, for whatever reason, you feel you need a little more help in the food area, then get hold of the bestseller *Freedom from the Diet Trap: Slim for Life*. I have such a passion for my first book and I think everyone should read it. Despite the title, it is not simply for people battling with the bulge – it is for anyone who eats food. If you have any other addiction problems please come and see us at one of our retreats.

In case we never get to meet, enjoy your freedom and make your life extraordinary.

Chocs Away!
Jason Vale